American Medical Association

Physicians dedicated to the health of America

Council on Ethical and Judicial Affairs

Code of Medical Ethics

Current Opinions

2000–2001 Edition

Copies of the annotated version (product number OP632300) may be ordered from:
Order Department
American Medical Association
515 N State Street
Chicago, IL 60610
800 621-8335

ISBN 1-57947-152-8

ES31:00-283:1.5M:6/00

Contents

1.00 Introduction

2.00 Opinions on Social Policy Issues

3.00   Opinions on Interprofessional Relations

4.00   Opinions on Hospital Relations

5.00   Opinions on Confidentiality, Advertising, and Communications Media Relations

6.00   Opinions on Fees and Charges

7.00   Opinions on Physician Records

8.00   Opinions on Practice Matters

9.00   Opinions on Professional Rights and Responsibilities

10.00   Opinions on the Patient-Physician Relationship

Appendix

Index

Preface

This edition of *Current Opinions* of the Council on Ethical and Judicial Affairs replaces all previous editions of *Current Opinions* and includes opinions based on reports adopted through June 1999. It is one component of the American Medical Association's Code of Ethics; the other components are the Principles of Medical Ethics, Fundamental Elements of the Patient-Physician Relationship, and the Reports of the Council on Ethical and Judicial Affairs. The Principles and Fundamental Elements precede the opinions in this volume. Reports are published separately.

The Principles of Medical Ethics are the primary component of the Code. They establish the core ethical principles from which the other components of the Code are derived. The Principles were most recently revised in 1980.

Fundamental Elements of the Patient-Physician Relationship enunciates the basic rights to which patients are entitled from their physicians.

Current Opinions reflects the application of the Principles of Medical Ethics to more than 160 specific ethical issues in medicine, including health care rationing, genetic testing, withdrawal of life-sustaining treatment, and family violence. Much as courts of law elaborate on constitutional principles in their holdings, the Council develops the meaning of the Principles of Medical Ethics in its opinions. Accordingly, each opinion is followed by one or more roman numerals that identify the Principle(s) from which the opinion is derived.

An annotated version of *Current Opinions* is also available which includes citations to the opinion in judicial rulings and the medical, ethical, and legal literature.

The Reports—from which many of the opinions are derived—discuss the rationale behind the Council's opinions, providing a detailed analysis of the relevant ethical considerations.

All four components of the AMA's Code of Ethics need to be consulted to determine the Association's positions on ethical issues. In addition, the AMA's House of Delegates at times issues statements on ethical issues. These statements are contained in the AMA's electronic policy database, the *PolicyFinder*. Because the Council on Ethical and Judicial Affairs is responsible for determining the AMA's positions on ethical issues, statements by the House of Delegates should be construed as the view of the House of Delegates but not as the ethics policy of the Association.

Medical ethics involve the professional responsibilities and obligations of physicians. Behavior relating to medical etiquette or custom is not addressed in *Current Opinions*. The opinions which follow are intended as guides to responsible professional behavior.

No one Principle of Medical Ethics can stand alone or be individually applied to a situation. In all instances, it is the overall intent and influence of the Principles of Medical Ethics which shall measure ethical behavior for the physician. Council opinions are issued under its authority to interpret the

Principles of Medical Ethics and to investigate general ethical conditions and all matters pertaining to the relations of physicians to one another and to the public.

The Council on Ethical and Judicial Affairs encourages comments and suggestions for future editions of this publication.

Council on Ethical and Judicial Affairs

1998-1999

Robert M. Tenery, Jr., MD, Chair

Herbert Rakatansky, MD, Vice Chair

Michael S. Goldrich, MD

John C. Madden, III

Leonard J. Morse, MD

John M. O'Bannon, III, MD

Frank A. Riddick, Jr., MD

Victoria N. Ruff, MD

Sherie Smalley, MD

1999-2000

Herbert Rakatansky, MD, Chair

Frank A. Riddick, Jr., MD, Vice Chair

Michael S. Goldrich, MD

Leonard J. Morse, MD

John M. O'Bannon, III, MD

Priscilla Ray, MD

Sherie Smalley, MD

Robert M. Tenery, Jr., MD

Matthew Weiss

Linda L. Emanuel, MD, PhD, Vice President, Ethics Standards

Audiey C. Kao, MD, PhD, Assist. Vice President, Ethics Standards

Jessica Berg, JD, Council Secretary

Karine Morin, LLM, Council Secretary

Alex J. Krasny, Staff Associate

Andrew H. Maixner, Staff Associate

Blaire S. Osgood, Senior Staff Associate

Samuel C. Seiden, Staff Associate

E. Ratcliffe Anderson, Jr., MD,
   Executive Vice President/Chief Executive Officer

Reed V. Tuckson, MD, Senior Vice President, Professional Standards

History

The Oath of Hippocrates, a brief statement of principles, has come down through history as a living statement of ideals to be cherished by the physician. This Oath was conceived some time during the period of Grecian greatness, probably in the fifth century B.C. It protected rights of the patient and appealed to the inner and finer instincts of the physician without imposing sanctions or penalties on him or her. Other civilizations subsequently developed written principles, but the Oath of Hippocrates (Christianized in the tenth or eleventh century A.D. to eliminate reference to pagan gods) has remained in Western Civilization as an expression of ideal conduct for the physician.

The most significant contribution to Western medical ethical history subsequent to Hippocrates was made by Thomas Percival, an English physician, philosopher, and writer. In 1803, he published his Code of Medical Ethics. His personality, his interest in sociological matters, and his close association with the Manchester Infirmary led to the preparation of a scheme of professional conduct relative to hospitals and other charities from which he drafted the code that bears his name.

At the first official meeting of the American Medical Association at Philadelphia in 1847, the two principal items of business were the establishment of a code of ethics and the creation of minimum requirements for medical education and training. Although the Medical Society of the State of New York and the Medico-Chirurgical Society of Baltimore had formal written codes of medical ethics prior to this time, it is clear the AMA's first adopted Code of Ethics was based on Percival's Code.

In general, the language and concepts of the original Code adopted by the Association in 1847 remained the same throughout the years. There were revisions, of course, which reflected the temper of the times and the eternal quest to express basic concepts with clarity. Major revisions did occur in 1903, 1912, 1947, and 1994.

In December 1955, an attempt was made to distinguish medical ethics from matters of etiquette. A draft of a two-part code seeking to accomplish this was submitted to the House of Delegates at that time but was not accepted. This proposal was, in effect, a separation of then existing statements found in the Principles into two categories. Little or no change was made in the language of the 48 sections of the Principles.

Subsequently, in June 1956, a seemingly radical proposal was submitted to the House of Delegates for consideration. This proposal, a short version of the Principles, was discussed at the December 1956 session of the House after wide publication and broad consideration among members of the medical profession. It was postponed for final consideration until the June 1957 meeting of the House of Delegates, when the short version was adopted.

The format of the Principles adopted in June 1957 is a change from the format of the Principles promulgated by Percival in 1803 and accepted by the Association in 1847. Ten short sections, preceded by a preamble, succinctly express the fundamental concepts embodied in the present (1955) Principles, according to the report of the Council on Constitution and Bylaws. That Council assured the House of Delegates in its June 1957 report that "every basic principle has been preserved; on the other hand, as much as possible of the prolixity and ambiguity which in the past obstructed ready explanation, practical codification and particular selection of basic concepts has been eliminated."

In 1977, the Judicial Council recommended to the House of Delegates that the AMA Principles of Medical Ethics be revised to clarify and update the language, to eliminate reference to gender, and to seek a proper and reasonable balance between professional standards and contemporary legal standards in our changing society. Given the desire of the Judicial Council for a new version of the Principles to be widely accepted and accurately understood, in 1978 the Judicial Council recommended that a special committee of the House be appointed to consider such a revision. This was done in 1980, and the House of Delegates adopted the revision of the AMA Principles of Medical Ethics at its Annual Meeting in June 1980.

In June 1985, the Judicial Council became the Council on Ethical and Judicial Affairs.

American Medical Association
Principles of Medical Ethics

Preamble:

The medical profession has long subscribed to a body of ethical statements developed primarily for the benefit of the patient. As a member of this profession, a physician must recognize responsibility not only to patients, but also to society, to other health professionals, and to self. The following Principles adopted by the American Medical Association are not laws, but standards of conduct which define the essentials of honorable behavior for the physician.

I. A physician shall be dedicated to providing competent medical service with compassion and respect for human dignity.

II. A physician shall deal honestly with patients and colleagues, and strive to expose those physicians deficient in character or competence, or who engage in fraud or deception.

III. A physician shall respect the law and also recognize a responsibility to seek changes in those requirements which are contrary to the best interests of the patient.

IV. A physician shall respect the rights of patients, of colleagues, and of other health professionals, and shall safeguard patient confidences within the constraints of the law.

V. A physician shall continue to study, apply and advance scientific knowledge, make relevant information available to patients, colleagues, and the public, obtain consultation, and use the talents of other health professionals when indicated.

VI. A physician shall, in the provision of appropriate patient care, except in emergencies, be free to choose whom to serve, with whom to associate, and the environment in which to provide medical services.

VII. A physician shall recognize a responsibility to participate in activities contributing to an improved community.

Fundamental Elements of the Patient-Physician Relationship

From ancient times, physicians have recognized that the health and well-being of patients depends upon a collaborative effort between physician and patient. Patients share with physicians the responsibility for their own health care. The patient-physician relationship is of greatest benefit to patients when they bring medical problems to the attention of their physicians in a timely fashion, provide information about their medical condition to the best of their ability, and work with their physicians in a mutually respectful alliance. Physicians can best contribute to this alliance by serving as their patients' advocate and by fostering these rights:

1. The patient has the right to receive information from physicians and to discuss the benefits, risks, and costs of appropriate treatment alternatives. Patients should receive guidance from their physicians as to the optimal course of action. Patients are also entitled to obtain copies or summaries of their medical records, to have their questions answered, to be advised of potential conflicts of interest that their physicians might have, and to receive independent professional opinions.

2. The patient has the right to make decisions regarding the health care that is recommended by his or her physician. Accordingly, patients may accept or refuse any recommended medical treatment.

3. The patient has the right to courtesy, respect, dignity, responsiveness, and timely attention to his or her needs.

4. The patient has the right to confidentiality. The physician should not reveal confidential communications or information without the consent of the patient, unless provided for by law or by the need to protect the welfare of the individual or the public interest.

5. The patient has the right to continuity of health care. The physician has an obligation to cooperate in the coordination of medically indicated care with other health care providers treating the patient. The physician may not discontinue treatment of a patient as long as further treatment is medically indicated, without giving the patient reasonable assistance and sufficient opportunity to make alternative arrangements for care.

6. The patient has a basic right to have available adequate health care. Physicians, along with the rest of society, should continue to work toward this goal. Fulfillment of this right is dependent on society providing resources so that no patient is deprived of necessary care because of an inability to pay for the care. Physicians should continue their traditional assumption of a part of the responsibility for the medical care of those who cannot afford essential health care. Physicians should advocate for patients in dealing with third parties when appropriate.

Issued June 1992 based on the report "Fundamental Elements of the Patient-Physician Relationship," adopted June 1990.

Updated 1993.

1.00 Introduction

1.01 Terminology

The term "ethical" is used in opinions of the Council on Ethical and Judicial Affairs to refer to matters involving (1) moral principles or practices and (2) matters of social policy involving issues of morality in the practice of medicine. The term "unethical" is used to refer to professional conduct which fails to conform to these moral standards or policies.

Many of the Council's opinions lay out specific duties and obligations for physicians. Violation of these principles and opinions represents unethical conduct and may justify disciplinary action such as censure, suspension, or expulsion from medical society membership.

Issued prior to April 1977.

Updated June 1994 and June 1996.

1.02 The Relation of Law and Ethics

The following statements are intended to clarify the relationship between law and ethics.

Ethical values and legal principles are usually closely related, but ethical obligations typically exceed legal duties. In some cases, the law mandates unethical conduct. In general, when physicians believe a law is unjust, they should work to change the law. In exceptional circumstances of unjust laws, ethical responsibilities should supersede legal obligations.

The fact that a physician charged with allegedly illegal conduct is acquitted or exonerated in civil or criminal proceedings does not necessarily mean that the physician acted ethically.

Issued prior to April 1977.

Updated June 1994.

2.00 Opinions on Social Policy Issues

2.01 Abortion

The Principles of Medical Ethics of the AMA do not prohibit a physician from performing an abortion in accordance with good medical practice and under circumstances that do not violate the law. (III, IV)

Issued prior to April 1977.

2.015 Mandatory Parental Consent to Abortion

Physicians should ascertain the law in their state on parental involvement to ensure that their procedures are consistent with their legal obligations.

Physicians should strongly encourage minors to discuss their pregnancy with their parents. Physicians should explain how parental involvement can be helpful and that parents are generally very understanding and supportive. If a minor expresses concerns about parental involvement, the physician should ensure that the minor's reluctance is not based on any misperceptions about the likely consequences of parental involvement.

Physicians should not feel or be compelled to require minors to involve their parents before deciding whether to undergo an abortion. The patient, even an adolescent, generally must decide whether, on balance, parental involvement is advisable. Accordingly, minors should ultimately be allowed to decide whether parental involvement is appropriate. Physicians should explain under what circumstances (e.g., life-threatening emergency) the minor's confidentiality will need to be abrogated.

Physicians should try to ensure that minor patients have made an informed decision after giving careful consideration to the issues involved. They should encourage their minor patients to consult alternative sources if parents are not going to be involved in the abortion decision. Minors should be urged to seek the advice and counsel of those adults in whom they have confidence, including professional counselors, relatives, friends, teachers, or the clergy. (III, IV)

Issued June 1994 based on the report "Mandatory Parental Consent to Abortion," adopted June 1992. (JAMA. 1993; 269: 82-86)

2.02   Abuse of Spouses, Children, Elderly Persons, and Others at Risk

The following are guidelines for detecting and treating family violence:

Due to the prevalence and medical consequences of family violence, physicians should routinely inquire about physical, sexual, and psychological abuse as part of the medical history. Physicians must also consider abuse in the differential diagnosis for a number of medical complaints, particularly when treating women.

Physicians who are likely to have the opportunity to detect abuse in the course of their work have an obligation to familiarize themselves with protocols for diagnosing and treating abuse and with community resources for battered women, children and elderly persons.

Physicians also have a duty to be aware of societal misconceptions about abuse and prevent these from affecting the diagnosis and management of abuse. Such misconceptions include the belief that abuse is a rare occurrence; that abuse does not occur in "normal" families; that abuse is a private problem best resolved without outside interference; and that victims are responsible for the abuse.

In order to improve physician knowledge of family violence, physicians must be better trained to identify signs of abuse and to work cooperatively with the range of community services currently involved. Hospitals should require additional training for those physicians who are likely to see victims of abuse. Comprehensive training on family violence should be required in medical school curricula and in residency programs for specialties in which family violence is likely to be encountered.

The following are guidelines for the reporting of abuse:

Laws that require the reporting of cases of suspected abuse of children and elderly persons often create a difficult dilemma for the physician. The parties involved, both the suspected offenders and the victims, will often plead with the physician that the matter be kept confidential and not be disclosed or reported for investigation by public authorities.

Children who have been seriously injured, apparently by their parents, may nevertheless try to protect their parents by saying that the injuries were caused by an accident, such as a fall. The reason may stem from the natural parent-child relationship or fear of further punishment. Even institutionalized elderly patients who have been physically maltreated may be concerned that disclosure of what has occurred might lead to further and more drastic maltreatment by those responsible.

The physician should comply with the laws requiring reporting of suspected cases of abuse of spouses, children, elderly persons, and others.

Public officials concerned with the welfare of children and elderly persons have expressed the opinion that the incidence of physical violence to these persons is rapidly increasing and that a very substantial percentage of such cases is unreported by hospital personnel and physicians. A child or elderly person brought to a physician with a suspicious injury is the patient whose interests require the protection of law in a particular situation, even though the physician may also provide services from time to time to parents or other members of the family.

3

The obligation to comply with statutory requirements is clearly stated in the Principles of Medical Ethics. Absent such legal requirement, for mentally competent, adult victims of abuse, physicians should not report to state authorities without the consent of the patient. Physicians, however, do have an ethical obligation to intervene. Actions should include, but would not be limited to: suggesting the possibility of abuse with the adult patient, discussing the safety mechanisms available to the adult patient (e.g. reporting to the police or appropriate state authority), making available to the adult patient a list of community and legal resources, providing ongoing support, and documenting the situation for future reference. Physicians must discuss possible interventions and the problem of family violence with adult patients in privacy and safety. (I, III)

Issued December 1982.

Updated June 1994 based on the report "Physicians and Family Violence: Ethical Considerations," adopted December 1991 (JAMA. 1992; 267: 3190-3193); updated June 1996; and updated June 2000 based on the report "Domestic Violence Intervention," adopted June 1998.

2.03   Allocation of Limited Medical Resources

A physician has a duty to do all that he or she can for the benefit of the individual patient. Policies for allocating limited resources have the potential to limit the ability of physicians to fulfill this obligation to patients. Physicians have a responsibility to participate and to contribute their professional expertise in order to safeguard the interests of patients in decisions made at the societal level regarding the allocation or rationing of health resources.

Decisions regarding the allocation of limited medical resources among patients should consider only ethically appropriate criteria relating to medical need. These criteria include likelihood of benefit, urgency of need, change in quality of life, duration of benefit, and, in some cases, the amount of resources required for successful treatment. In general, only very substantial differences among patients are ethically relevant; the greater the disparities, the more justified the use of these criteria becomes. In making quality of life judgments, patients should first be prioritized so that death or extremely poor outcomes are avoided; then, patients should be prioritized according to change in quality of life, but only when there are very substantial differences among patients. Non-medical criteria, such as ability to pay, age, social worth, perceived obstacles to treatment, patient contribution to illness, or past use of resources should not be considered.

Allocation decisions should respect the individuality of patients and the particulars of individual cases as much as possible. When very substantial differences do not exist among potential recipients of treatment on the basis of the appropriate criteria defined above, a "first-come-first-served" approach or some other equal opportunity mechanism should be employed to make final allocation decisions. Though there are several ethically acceptable strategies for implementing these criteria, no single strategy is ethically mandated. Acceptable approaches include a three-tiered system, a minimal threshold approach, and a weighted formula. Decision-making mechanisms should be objective, flexible, and consistent to ensure that all patients are treated equally.

The treating physician must remain a patient advocate and therefore should not make allocation decisions. Patients denied access to resources have the right to be informed of the reasoning behind the decision. The allocation procedures of institutions controlling scarce resources should be disclosed to the public as well as subject to regular peer review from the medical profession. (I,VII)

Issued March 1981.

Updated June 1994 based on the report "Ethical Considerations in the Allocation of Organs and Other Scarce Medical Resources Among Patients," adopted June 1993 (*Arch Intern Med.* 1995; 155: 29-40).

2.035   Futile Care

Physicians are not ethically obligated to deliver care that, in their best professional judgment, will not have a reasonable chance of benefiting their patients. Patients should not be given treatments simply because they demand them. Denial of treatment should be justified by reliance on openly stated ethical principles and acceptable standards of care, as defined in Opinions 2.03 and 2.095, not on the concept of "futility," which cannot be meaningfully defined. (I, IV)

Issued June 1994.

2.037   Medical Futility in End-of-Life Care

When further intervention to prolong the life of a patient becomes futile, physicians have an obligation to shift the intent of care toward comfort and closure. However, there are necessary value judgments involved in coming to the assessment of futility. These judgments must give consideration to patient or proxy assessments of worthwhile outcome. They should also take into account the physician or other provider's perception of intent in treatment, which should not be to prolong the dying process without benefit to the patient or to others with legitimate interests. They may also take into account community and institutional standards, which in turn may have used physiological or functional outcome measures.

Nevertheless, conflicts between the parties may persist in determining what is futility in the particular instance. This may interrupt satisfactory decision-making and adversely affect patient care, family satisfaction, and physician-clinical team functioning. To assist in fair and satisfactory decision-making about what constitutes futile intervention:

(1) All health care institutions, whether large or small, should adopt a policy on medical futility; and

(2) Policies on medical futility should follow a due process approach. The following seven steps should be included in such a due process approach to declaring futility in specific cases.

   (a) Earnest attempts should be made in advance to deliberate over and negotiate prior understandings between patient, proxy and physician on what constitutes futile care for the patient, and what falls within acceptable limits for the physician, family, and possibly also the institution.

(b) Joint decision-making should occur between patient or proxy and physician to the maximum extent possible.

(c) Attempts should be made to negotiate disagreements if they arise, and to reach resolution within all parties' acceptable limits, with the assistance of consultants as appropriate.

(d) Involvement of an institutional committee such as the ethics committee should be requested if disagreements are irresolvable.

(e) If the institutional review supports the patient's position and the physician remains unpersuaded, transfer of care to another physician within the institution may be arranged.

(f) If the process supports the physician's position and the patient/proxy remains unpersuaded, transfer to another institution may be sought and, if done, should be supported by the transferring and receiving institution.

(g) If transfer is not possible, the intervention need not be offered.

Issued June 1997 based on the report "Medical Futility in End-of-Life Care," adopted December 1996.

2.04   The previous Opinion 2.04, **Artificial Insemination by Known Donor**, issued prior to April 1977, was replaced by the current Opinion 2.04.

2.04   Artificial Insemination by Known Donor

Any individual or couple contemplating artificial insemination by husband, partner, or other known donor should be counseled about the full range of infectious and genetic diseases for which the donor or recipient can be screened, including HIV infection. Full medical history disclosure and appropriate diagnostic screening should be recommended to the donor and recipient but are not required.

Informed consent for artificial insemination should include disclosure of risks, benefits, and likely success rate of the method proposed and potential alternative methods. Individuals should receive information about screening, costs, and procedures for confidentiality, when applicable. The prospective parents or parent should be informed of the laws regarding the rights of children conceived by artificial insemination, as well as the laws regarding parental rights and obligations. If the donor is married to the recipient, resultant children will have all the rights of a child conceived naturally.

If the donor and recipient are not married, an appropriate legal rule would treat the situation as if the donor were anonymous: the recipient would be considered the sole parent of the child except in cases where both donor and recipient agree to recognize a paternity right.

Sex selection of sperm for the purposes of avoiding a sex-linked inheritable disease is appropriate. However, physicians should not participate in sex selection for reasons of gender preference. Physicians should encourage a prospective parent or parents to consider the value of both sexes.

If semen is frozen and the donor dies before it is used, the frozen semen should not be used or donated for purposes other than those originally intended by the donor. If the donor left no instructions, it is reasonable to allow the remaining partner to use the semen for artificial insemination but not to donate it to someone else. However, the donor should be advised of such a policy at the time of donation and be given an opportunity to override it. (I, V)

Issued June 1993.

2.05   The previous Opinion 2.05, **Artificial Insemination by Donor**, issued 1983, was replaced by the current Opinion 2.05.

2.05   Artificial Insemination by Anonymous Donor

Thorough medical histories must be taken of all candidates for anonymous semen donation. All potential donors must also be screened for infectious or inheritable diseases which could adversely affect the recipient or the resultant child. Frozen semen should be used for artificial insemination because it enables the donor to be tested for HIV infection at the time of donation, and again after an interval before the original semen is used, thus increasing the likelihood that the semen is free of HIV infection. Physicians should rely on the guidelines formulated by relevant professional organizations, such as the American Society of Reproductive Medicine, the Centers for Disease Control and Prevention, and the Food and Drug Administration, in determining the interval between the initial and final HIV test, which disorders to screen for, and which procedures to use in screening.

Physicians should maintain a permanent record which includes both identifying and non-identifying health and genetic screening information. Other than exceptional situations where identifying information may be required, physicians should release only non-identifying health related information in order to preserve the confidentiality of the semen donor. Physicians should maintain permanent records of donors to fulfill the following obligations: (1) to exclude individuals from the donor pool who test positive for infectious or inheritable diseases, (2) to limit the number of pregnancies resulting from a single donor source so as to avoid future consanguineous marriages or reproduction, (3) to notify donors of screening results which indicate the presence of an infectious or inheritable disease, and (4) to notify donors if a child born through artificial insemination has a disorder which may have been transmitted by the donor.

Informed consent for artificial insemination should include disclosure of risks, benefits, likely success rate of the method proposed and potential alternative methods, and costs. Both recipients and donors should be informed of the reasons for screening and confidentiality. They should also know the extent of access to non-identifying and identifying information about the donor. Participants should be advised to consider the legal ramifications, if any, of artificial insemination by anonymous donor.

The consent of the husband is ethically appropriate if he is to become the legal father of the resultant child from artificial insemination by anonymous donor. Anonymous donors cannot assume the rights or responsibilities of parenthood for children born through therapeutic donor insemination, nor should they be required to assume them.

In the case of single women or women who are part of a homosexual couple, it is not unethical to provide artificial insemination as a reproductive option.

Sex selection of sperm for the purposes of avoiding a sex-linked inheritable disease is appropriate. However, physicians should not participate in sex selection of sperm for reasons of gender preference. Physicians should encourage a prospective parent or parents to consider the value of both sexes.

In general, it is inappropriate to offer compensation to donors to encourage donation over and above reimbursement for time and actual expenses. (I, V)

Issued June 1993.

2.055   Ethical Conduct in Assisted Reproductive Technology

The following guidelines are intended to emphasize the value of existing standards to ensure ethical practices in assisted reproductive technology (ART):

The medical professions' development of technical and ethical guidelines for ART should continue. Education of the profession and patients should be pursued through widely disseminated information. Such material should include information on clinic-specific success rates.

Fertility laboratories not currently participating in a credible professional accreditation program are encouraged to do so. Professional self-regulation is also encouraged through signed pledges to meet established ethical standards and to comply with laboratory accreditation efforts. Physicians who become aware of unethical practices must report such conduct to the appropriate body. Physicians also should be willing to provide expert testimony when needed. Specialty societies should discuss the development of mechanisms for disciplinary action, such as revocation of membership, for members who fail to comply with ethical standards.

Patients should be fully informed about all aspects of ART applicable to their particular clinical profile. A well-researched, validated informed consent instrument would be useful for the benefit of patients and professionals. Payment based on clinical outcome is unacceptable.

Physicians and clinicians practicing ART should use accurate descriptors of available services, success rates, and fee structure and payment obligations in promotional materials.

If legislation on regulation of ART laboratories, advertising practices, or related issues is adopted, it should include adequate financial resources to ensure the intended action can be implemented. Improved legislative protection may be needed to protect physicians and their professional organizations when they provide testimony on unethical conduct of colleagues. (I, V)

Issued December 1998 based on the report "Issues of Ethical Conduct in Assisted Reproductive Technology," adopted June 1996.

2.06 Capital Punishment

An individual's opinion on capital punishment is the personal moral decision of the individual. A physician, as a member of a profession dedicated to preserving life when there is hope of doing so, should not be a participant in a legally authorized execution. Physician participation in execution is defined generally as actions which would fall into one or more of the following categories: (1) an action which would directly cause the death of the condemned; (2) an action which would assist, supervise, or contribute to the ability of another individual to directly cause the death of the condemned; (3) an action which could automatically cause an execution to be carried out on a condemned prisoner.

Physician participation in an execution includes, but is not limited to, the following actions: prescribing or administering tranquilizers and other psychotropic agents and medications that are part of the execution procedure; monitoring vital signs on site or remotely (including monitoring electrocardiograms); attending or observing an execution as a physician; and rendering of technical advice regarding execution.

In the case where the method of execution is lethal injection, the following actions by the physician would also constitute physician participation in execution: selecting injection sites; starting intravenous lines as a port for a lethal injection device; prescribing, preparing, administering, or supervising injection drugs or their doses or types; inspecting, testing, or maintaining lethal injection devices; and consulting with or supervising lethal injection personnel.

The following actions do not constitute physician participation in execution: (1) testifying as to medical history and diagnoses or mental state as they relate to competence to stand trial, testifying as to relevant medical evidence during trial, testifying as to medical aspects of aggravating or mitigating circumstances during the penalty phase of a capital case, or testifying as to medical diagnoses as they relate to the legal assessment of competence for execution; (2) certifying death, provided that the condemned has been declared dead by another person; (3) witnessing an execution in a totally nonprofessional capacity; (4) witnessing an execution at the specific voluntary request of the condemned person, provided that the physician observes the execution in a nonprofessional capacity; and (5) relieving the acute suffering of a condemned person while awaiting execution, including providing tranquilizers at the specific voluntary request of the condemned person to help relieve pain or anxiety in anticipation of the execution.

Physicians should not determine legal competence to be executed. A physician's medical opinion should be merely one aspect of the information taken into account by a legal decision maker such as a judge or hearing officer. When a condemned prisoner has been declared incompetent to be executed, physicians should not treat the prisoner for the purpose of restoring competence unless a commutation order is issued before treatment begins. The task of re-evaluating the prisoner should be performed by an independent physician examiner. If the incompetent prisoner is undergoing extreme suffering as a result of psychosis or any other illness, medical intervention intended to mitigate the level of suffering is ethically permissible. No physician should be compelled to participate in the process of establishing a prisoner's competence or be involved with treatment of an incompetent, condemned prisoner if such activity is contrary to the physician's personal beliefs. Under those circumstances, physicians should be permitted to transfer care of the prisoner to another physician.

Organ donation by condemned prisoners is permissible only if (1) the decision to donate was made before the prisoner's conviction, (2) the donated tissue is harvested after the prisoner has been pronounced dead and the body removed from the death chamber, and (3) physicians do not provide advice on modifying the method of execution for any individual to facilitate donation. (I)

Issued July 1980.

Updated June 1994 based on the report "Physician Participation in Capital Punishment," adopted December 1992 (JAMA. 1993; 270: 365-368); updated June 1996 based on the report "Physician Participation in Capital Punishment: Evaluations of Prisoner Competence to be Executed; Treatment to Restore Competence to be Executed," adopted in June 1995; updated December 1999; and updated June 2000 based on the report "Defining Physician Participation in State Executions," adopted June 1998.

2.065   Court-Initiated Medical Treatments in Criminal Cases

Physicians can ethically participate in court-initiated medical treatments only if the procedure being mandated is therapeutically efficacious and is therefore undoubtedly not a form of punishment or solely a mechanism of social control. While a court has the authority to identify criminal behavior, a court does not have the ability to make a medical diagnosis or to determine the type of treatment that will be administered. In accordance with ethical practice, physicians should treat patients based on sound medical diagnoses, not court defined behaviors. This is particularly important where the treatment involves inpatient therapy, surgical intervention, or pharmacological treatment. In these cases, diagnosis can be made initially by the physician who will do the treatment, but must then be confirmed by an independent physician or a panel of physicians not responsible to the state. A second opinion is not necessary in cases of court-ordered counseling or referrals for psychiatric evaluations.

A recognized, authoritative medical body, such as a national specialty society, should pre-establish scientifically valid treatments for medically determined diagnoses. Such pre-established acceptable treatments should then be applied on a case by case basis.

The physician who will perform the treatment must be able to conclude, in good conscience and to the best of his or her professional judgment, that the informed consent was given voluntarily to the extent possible, recognizing the element of coercion that is inevitably present. In cases involving in-patient therapy, surgical intervention, or pharmacological treatment, an independent physician or a panel of physicians not responsible to the state should confirm that the informed consent was given in accordance with these guidelines. (I, III)

Issued December 1998 based on the report "Court-Initiated Medical Treatment in Criminal Cases," adopted June 1998.

2.067 Torture

Torture refers to the deliberate, systematic or wanton administration of cruel, inhumane and degrading treatments or punishments during imprisonment or detainment.

Physicians must oppose and must not participate in torture for any reason. Participation in torture includes, but is not limited to, providing or withholding any services, substances or knowledge to facilitate the practice of torture. Physicians must not be present when torture is used or threatened.

Physicians may treat prisoners or detainees if doing so is in their best interest, but physicians should not treat individuals to verify their health so that torture can begin or continue. Physicians who treat torture victims should not be persecuted. Physicians should help provide support for victims of torture and, whenever possible, strive to change situations in which torture is practiced or the potential for torture is great. (I, III)

Issued December 1999.

2.07 Clinical Investigation

The following guidelines are intended to aid physicians in fulfilling their ethical responsibilities when they engage in the clinical investigation of new drugs and procedures.

(1) A physician may participate in clinical investigation only to the extent that those activities are a part of a systematic program competently designed, under accepted standards of scientific research, to produce data which are scientifically valid and significant.

(2) In conducting clinical investigation, the investigator should demonstrate the same concern and caution for the welfare, safety, and comfort of the person involved as is required of a physician who is furnishing medical care to a patient independent of any clinical investigation.

(3) Minors or mentally incompetent persons may be used as subjects in clinical investigation only if:
   (a) The nature of the investigation is such that mentally competent adults would not be suitable subjects.
   (b) Consent, in writing, is given by a legally authorized representative of the subject under circumstances in which informed and prudent adults would reasonably be expected to volunteer themselves or their children as subjects.

(4) In clinical investigation primarily for treatment:
   (a) The physician must recognize that the patient-physician relationship exists and that professional judgment and skill must be exercised in the best interest of the patient.
   (b) Voluntary written consent must be obtained from the patient, or from the patient's legally authorized representative if the patient lacks the capacity to consent, following: (a) disclosure that the physician intends to use an investigational drug or experimental procedure, (b) a reasonable explanation of the nature of the drug or procedure to be used, risks

to be expected, and possible therapeutic benefits, (c) an offer to answer any inquiries concerning the drug or procedure, and (d) a disclosure of alternative drugs or procedures that may be available. Physicians should be completely objective in discussing the details of the drug or procedure to be employed, the pain and discomfort that may be anticipated, known risks and possible hazards, the quality of life to be expected, and particularly the alternatives. Especially, physicians should not use persuasion to obtain consent which otherwise might not be forthcoming, nor should expectations be encouraged beyond those which the circumstances reasonably and realistically justify.

    (i) In exceptional circumstances, where the experimental treatment is the only potential treatment for the patient and full disclosure of information concerning the nature of the drug or experimental procedure or risks would pose such a serious psychological threat of detriment to the patient as to be medically contraindicated, such information may be withheld from the patient. In these circumstances, such information should be disclosed to a responsible relative or friend of the patient where possible.

    (ii) Ordinarily, consent should be in writing, except where the physician deems it necessary to rely upon consent in other than written form because of the physical or emotional state of the patient.

(5) In clinical investigation primarily for the accumulation of scientific knowledge:

    (a) Adequate safeguards must be provided for the welfare, safety and comfort of the subject. It is fundamental social policy that the advancement of scientific knowledge must always be secondary to primary concern for the individual.

    (b) Consent, in writing, should be obtained from the subject, or from a legally authorized representative if the subject lacks the capacity to consent, following: (a) disclosure of the fact that an investigational drug or procedure is to be used, (b) a reasonable explanation of the nature of the procedure to be used and risks to be expected, and (c) an offer to answer any inquiries concerning the drug or procedure.

(6) No person may be used as a subject in clinical investigation against his or her will.

(7) The overuse of institutionalized persons in research is an unfair distribution of research risks. Participation is coercive and not voluntary if the participant is subjected to powerful incentives and persuasion.

(8) The ultimate responsibility for the ethical conduct of science resides within the institution (academic, industrial, public, or private) which conducts scientific research and with the individual scientist. Research institutions should assure that rigorous scientific standards are upheld by each of their faculty, staff, and students and should extend these standards to all reports, publications, and databases produced by the institution. All medical schools and biomedical research institutions should implement guidelines for a review process for dealing with allegations of fraud. These guidelines should ensure that (a) the process used to resolve allegations of fraud does not damage science, (b) all parties are treated fairly and justly with a sensitivity to

reputations and vulnerabilities, (c) the highest degree of confidentiality is maintained, (d) the integrity of the process is maintained by an avoidance of real or apparent conflicts of interest, (e) resolution of charges is expeditious, (f) accurate and detailed documentation is kept throughout the process, and (g) responsibilities to all involved individuals, the public, research sponsors, the scientific literature, and the scientific community is met after resolution of charges. Academic institutions must be capable of, and committed to, implementing effective procedures for examining allegations of scientific fraud. No system of external monitoring should replace the efforts of an institution to set its own standards which fulfill its responsibility for the proper conduct of science and the training of scientists.

(9) With the approval of the patient or the patient's lawful representative, physicians should cooperate with the press and media to ensure that medical news concerning the progress of clinical investigation or the patient's condition is available more promptly and more accurately than would be possible without their assistance. On the other hand, the Council does not approve of practices designed to create fanfare, sensationalism to attract media attention, and unwarranted expressions of optimism because of short term progress, even though longer range prognosis is known from the beginning to be precarious. With the approval of the patient or the patient's family, the Council, however, encourages the objective disclosure to the press and media of pertinent information. If at all possible, the identity of the patient should remain confidential if the patient or the patient's family so desires. The situation should not be used for the commercial ends of participating physicians or the institutions involved. (I, III, V)

Issued prior to April 1977.

Updated June 1994 and June 1998.

2.071 Subject Selection for Clinical Trials

Ethical considerations in clinical research has traditionally focused on protecting research subjects. These protections may be especially important for those from socioeconomically diasdavantaged populations who may be more vulnerable to coercive pressures. The benefits from altruism that result from participation in research, particularly for severely chronically ill persons, may justify equitable consideration of historically disadvantaged populations such as the poor. With these considerations in mind, the following guidelines are offered:

Although the burdens of research should not fall disproportionately on socioeconomically disadvantaged populations, neither should such populations be categorically excluded, or discouraged, from research protocols.

Inclusion and exclusion criteria for a clinical study should be based on sound scientific principles. Conversely, participants in a clinical trial should be drawn from the qualifying population in the general geographic area of the trial without regard to race, ethnicity, economic status or gender.

If a subject's primary care physician determines that the subject received a clear medical benefit from the experimental intervention which is now moving towards marketing approval and chooses to seek authorization from the Food and Drug Administration (FDA) for continued use of the investigational therapy during the time period between the end of the protocol and the availability of the drug on the market, the investigator should work with the primary care physician, the product sponsor and the FDA to allow continued availability of the product. (I, V, VII)

Issued June 1998 based on the report "Subject Selection for Clinical Trials," adopted December 1997.

2.075 The Use of Placebo Controls in Clincal Trials

Placebo controls are an important part of medicine's commitment to ensuring that the safety and efficacy of new drugs are sufficiently established. Used appropriately, placebo controls can safely provide valuable data and should continue to be considered in the design of clinical trials. The existence of an accepted therapy does not necessarily preclude the use of such controls; however, physician-investigators should adhere to the following guidelines to ensure that the interests of patients who participate in clinical trials are protected.

(1) Investigators must be extremely thorough in obtaining informed consent from patients. To the extent that research is dependent upon the willingness of patients to accept a level of risk, their understanding of the potential harms involved must be a top priority of any clinical investigation. The possibility presented in some studies that patients often do not fully understand the research protocol and therefore truly can not give informed consent demonstrates a need to heighten the efforts of researchers to impress upon their subjects the nature of clinical research and the risks involved. Patients are capable of making decisions when presented with sufficient information and it is the responsibility of the institutional review board (IRB) and the individual investigators involved to ensure that each subject has been adequately informed and has given voluntary consent. Each patient must also be made aware that they can terminate their participation in a study at any time.

(2) Informed consent cannot be invoked to justify an inappropriate trial design. IRBs as well as investigators have an obligation to evaluate each study protocol to determine whether a placebo control is necessary and whether an alternative study design with another type of control would be sufficient for the purposes of research. Protocols that involve conditions causing death or irreversible damage cannot ethically employ a placebo control if alternative treatment would prevent or slow the illness progression. When studying illnesses characterized by severe or painful symptoms, investigators should thoroughly explore alternatives to the use of placebo controls. In general, the more severe the consequences and symptoms of the illness under study, the more difficult it will be to justify the use of a placebo control when alternative therapy exists. Consequently, there will almost certainly be conditions for which placebo controls cannot be justified. Similarly, the use of a placebo control will more easily be justified as the severity and number of negative side-effects of standard therapy increase.

(3) Researchers and IRBs should continue to minimize the amount of time patients are given placebo. The rationale provided by investigators for the

length of study will give IRBs the opportunity to ensure that patients are given placebo therapy for as short a time as possible to provide verifiable results. Additionally, the interim data analysis and monitoring currently in practice will allow researchers to terminate the study because of either positive or negative results, thus protecting patients from remaining on placebo unnecessarily. (I, V)

Issued June 1997 based on the report "Ethical Use of Placebo Controls in Clinical Trials," adopted June 1996.

2.08   The previous Opinion 2.08, **Clinical Investigation: Replacement of Vital Humans Organs**, issued July 1986, was deleted in 1994 and combined with Opinion 2.07.

2.08   Commercial Use of Human Tissue

The rapid growth of the biotechnology industry has resulted in the commercial availability of numerous therapeutic and other products developed from human tissue. Physicians contemplating the commercial use of human tissue should abide by the following guidelines:

(1) Informed consent must be obtained from patients for the use of organs or tissues in clinical research.

(2) Potential commercial applications must be disclosed to the patient before a profit is realized on products developed from biological materials.

(3) Human tissue and its products may not be used for commercial purposes without the informed consent of the patient who provided the original cellular material.

(4) Profits from the commercial use of human tissue and its products may be shared with patients, in accordance with lawful contractual agreements.

(5) The diagnostic and therapeutic alternatives offered to patients by their physicians should conform to standards of good medical practice and should not be influenced in any way by the commercial potential of the patient's tissue. (II, V)

Issued June 1994 based on the report "Who Should Profit from the Economic Value of Human Tissue? An Ethical Analysis," adopted June 1990.

2.09   Costs

While physicians should be conscious of costs and not provide or prescribe unnecessary services, concern for the quality of care the patient receives should be the physician's first consideration. This does not preclude the physician, individually or through medical or other organizations, from participating in policy-making with respect to social issues affecting health care. (I, VII)

Issued March 1981.

Updated June 1994 and June 1998.

2.095   The Provision of Adequate Health Care

Because society has an obligation to make access to an adequate level of health care available to all of its members regardless of ability to pay, physicians should contribute their expertise at a policy-making level to help achieve this goal. In determining whether particular procedures or treatments should be included in the adequate level of health care, the following ethical principles should be considered: (1) degree of benefit (the difference in outcome between treatment and no treatment), (2) likelihood of benefit, (3) duration of benefit, (4) cost, and (5) number of people who will benefit (referring to the fact that a treatment may benefit the patient and others who come into contact with the patient, as with a vaccination or antimicrobial drug).

Ethical principles require that a just process be used to determine the adequate level of health care. To ensure justice, the process for determining the adequate level of health care should include the following considerations: (1) democratic decision making with broad public input at both the developmental and final approval stages, (2) monitoring for variations in care that cannot be explained on medical grounds with special attention to evidence of discriminatory impact on historically disadvantaged groups, and (3) adjustment of the adequate level over time to ensure continued and broad public acceptance.

Because of the risk that inappropriate biases will influence the content of the basic benefits package, it may be desirable to avoid rigid or precise formulas to define the specific components of the basic benefits package. After applying the five ethical values listed above, it will be possible to designate some kinds of care as either clearly basic or clearly discretionary. However, for care that is not clearly basic or discretionary, seemingly objective formulas may result in choices that are inappropriately biased. For that care, therefore, it may be desirable to give equal consideration (e.g., through a process of random selection) to the different kinds of care when deciding which will be included in the basic benefits package. The mechanism for providing an adequate level of health care should ensure that the health care benefits for the poor will not be eroded over time. (VII)

Issued June 1994 based on the report "Ethical Issues in Health System Reform: The Provision of Adequate Health Care," adopted December 1993.

2.10   Fetal Research Guidelines

The following guidelines are offered as aids to physicians when they are engaged in fetal research:
(1) Physicians may participate in fetal research when their activities are part of a competently designed program, under accepted standards of scientific research, to produce data which are scientifically valid and significant.
(2) If appropriate, properly performed clinical studies on animals and non-gravid humans should precede any particular fetal research project.
(3) In fetal research projects, the investigator should demonstrate the same care and concern for the fetus as a physician providing fetal care or treatment in a non-research setting.

(4) All valid federal or state legal requirements should be followed.

(5) There should be no monetary payment to obtain any fetal material for fetal research projects.

(6) Competent peer review committees, review boards, or advisory boards should be available, when appropriate, to protect against the possible abuses that could arise in such research.

(7) Research on the so called dead fetus, macerated fetal material, fetal cells, fetal tissue, or fetal organs should be in accord with state laws on autopsy and state laws on organ transplantation or anatomical gifts.

(8) In fetal research primarily for treatment of the fetus:

    (a) Voluntary and informed consent, in writing, should be given by the gravid woman, acting in the best interest of the fetus.

    (b) Alternative treatment or methods of care, if any, should be carefully evaluated and fully explained. If simpler and safer treatment is available, it should be pursued.

(9) In research primarily for treatment of the gravid female:

    (a) Voluntary and informed consent, in writing, should be given by the patient.

    (b) Alternative treatment or methods of care should be carefully evaluated and fully explained to the patient. If simpler and safer treatment is available, it should be pursued.

    (c) If possible, the risk to the fetus should be the least possible, consistent with the gravid female's need for treatment.

(10) In fetal research involving a fetus in utero, primarily for the accumulation of scientific knowledge:

    (a) Voluntary and informed consent, in writing, should be given by the gravid woman under circumstances in which a prudent and informed adult would reasonably be expected to give such consent.

    (b) The risk to the fetus imposed by the research should be the least possible.

    (c) The purpose of research is the production of data and knowledge which are scientifically significant and which cannot otherwise be obtained.

    (d) In this area of research, it is especially important to emphasize that care and concern for the fetus should be demonstrated. (I, III, V)

Issued March 1980.

Updated June 1994.

2.105 Patenting the Human Genome

A patent grants the holder the right, for a limited amount of time, to prevent others from commercializing his or her inventions. At the same time, the patent system is designed to foster information sharing. Full disclosure of the invention—enabling another trained in the art to replicate it—is necessary to obtain a patent. Patenting is also thought to encourage private investment into research. Arguments have been made that the patenting of human genomic material sets a troubling precedent for the ownership or commodification of human life. DNA sequences, however, are not tantamount to human life, and it is unclear where and whether qualities uniquely human are found in genetic material.

Genetic research holds great potential for achieving new medical therapies. It remains unclear what role patenting will play in ensuring such development. At this time the Council concludes that granting patent protection should not hinder the goal of developing new beneficial technology and offers the following guidelines:

Patents on processes—for example, processes used to isolate and purify gene sequences, genes and proteins, or vehicles of gene therapy—do not raise the same ethical problems as patents on the substances themselves and are thus preferable.

Substance patents on purified proteins present fewer ethical problems than patents on genes or DNA sequences and are thus preferable.

Patent descriptions should be carefully constructed to ensure that the patent holder does not limit the use of a naturally occurring form of the substance in question. This includes patents on proteins, genes, and genetic sequences.

One of the goals of genetic research is to achieve better medical treatments and technologies. Granting patent protection should not hinder this goal. Individuals or entities holding patents on genetic material should not allow patents to languish and should negotiate and structure licensing agreements in such a way as to encourage the development of better medical technology. (V, VII)

Issued June 1998 based on the report "Patenting the Human Genome," adopted December 1997.

2.11   Gene Therapy

Gene therapy involves the replacement or modification of a genetic variant to restore or enhance cellular function or to improve the reaction of non-genetic therapies.

Two types of gene therapy have been identified: (1) somatic cell therapy, in which human cells other than germ cells are genetically altered, and (2) germ line therapy, in which a replacement gene is integrated into the genome of human gametes or their precursors, resulting in expression of the new gene in the patient's offspring and subsequent generations. The fundamental difference between germ line therapy and somatic cell therapy is that germ line therapy affects the welfare of subsequent generations and may be associated with increased risk and the potential for unpredictable and irreversible results. Because of the far-reaching implications of germ line therapy, it is appropriate to limit genetic intervention to somatic cells at this time.

The goal of both somatic cell and germ line therapy is to alleviate human suffering and disease by remedying disorders for which available therapies are not satisfactory. This goal should be pursued only within the ethical tradition of medicine, which gives primacy to the welfare of the patient whose safety and well-being must be vigorously protected. To the extent possible, experience with animal studies must be sufficient to assure the effectiveness and safety of the techniques used, and the predictability of the results.

Moreover, genetic manipulation generally should be utilized only for therapeutic purposes. Efforts to enhance "desirable" characteristics through the insertion of a modified or additional gene, or efforts to "improve" complex human traits—the eugenic development of offspring—are contrary not only to the ethical tradition of medicine, but also to the egalitarian values of our society. Because of the potential for abuse, genetic manipulation to affect non-disease traits may never be acceptable and perhaps should never be pursued. If it is ever allowed, at least three conditions would have to be met before it could be deemed ethically acceptable: (1) there would have to be a clear and meaningful benefit to the person, (2) there would have to be no trade-off with other characteristics or traits, and (3) all citizens would have to have equal access to the genetic technology, irrespective of income or other socioeconomic characteristics. These criteria should be viewed as a minimal, not an exhaustive, test of the ethical propriety of non-disease-related genetic intervention. As genetic technology and knowledge of the human genome develop further, additional guidelines may be required.

As gene therapy becomes feasible for a variety of human disorders, there are several practical factors to consider to ensure safe application of this technology in society. First, any gene therapy research should meet the Council's guidelines on clinical investigation (Opinion 2.07) and investigators must adhere to the standards of medical practice and professional responsibility. The proposed procedure must be fully discussed with the patient and the written informed consent of the patient or the patient's legal representative must be voluntary.

Investigators must be thorough in their attempts to eliminate any unwanted viral agents from the viral vector containing the corrective gene. The potential for adverse effects of the viral delivery system must be disclosed to the patient. The effectiveness of gene therapy must be evaluated fully, including the determination of the natural history of the disease and follow-up examination of subsequent generations. Gene therapy should be pursued only after the availablity or effectiveness of other possible therapies is found to be insufficient. These considerations should be reviewed, as appropriate, as procedures and scientific information develop. (I, V)

Issued December 1988.

Updated June 1994 based on the report "Prenatal Genetic Screeing," adopted December 1992 (*Arch Fam Med*. 1994; 2: 633-642), and updated June 1996.

2.12   Genetic Counseling

Three primary areas of prenatal genetic testing are: (1) screening or evaluating prospective parents for genetic disease before conception to predict the likelihood of conceiving an affected child; (2) analysis of a pre-embryo at the preimplantation stage of artificial reproductive techniques; and (3) in utero testing after conception, such as ultrasonography, amniocentesis, fetoscopy, and chorionic villus sampling, to determine the condition of the fetus. Physicians engaged in genetic counseling are ethically obligated to provide prospective parents with the basis for an informed decision for childbearing. Counseling should include reasons for and against testing as well as discussion of inappropriate uses of genetic testing. Prenatal genetic testing is most appropriate for women or couples whose medical histories or family backgrounds indicate an elevated risk of fetal genetic disorders. Women or couples without an elevated risk of genetic disease may legitimately request prenatal diagnosis, provided they understand and accept the risks involved. When counseling prospective parents, physicians should avoid the imposition of their personal moral values and the substitution of their own moral judgment for that of the prospective parents.

The physician should be aware that where a genetic defect is found in the fetus, prospective parents may request or refuse an abortion. Physicians who consider the legal and ethical requirements applicable to genetic counseling to be in conflict with their moral values and conscience may choose to limit their services to preconception diagnosis and advice or not provide any genetic services. However, the physician who is so disposed is nevertheless obligated to alert prospective parents when a potential genetic problem does exist, so that the patient may decide whether to seek further genetic counseling from another qualified specialist.

Genetic selection refers to the abortion or discard of a fetus or pre-embryo with a genetic abnormality. In general, it is ethically permissible for physicians to participate in genetic selection to prevent, cure, or treat genetic disease. However, selection to avoid a genetic disease may not always be appropriate, depending on factors such as the severity of the disease, the probability of its occurrence, the age at onset, and the time of gestation at which selection would occur. It would not be ethical to engage in selection on the basis of non-disease related characteristics or traits. (II, IV, V, VI)

Issued June 1983.

Updated June 1994 based on the report "Prenatal Genetic Screening," adopted December 1992 (*Arch Fam Med*. 1994; 3: 633-642).

2.13   Genetic Engineering

The Federal Recombinant DNA Advisors Committee and the Food and Drug Administration oversee and regulate gene splicing, recombinant DNA research, chemical synthesis of DNA molecules, and other genetic engineering research. However, for genetic engineering technologies that represent a significant departure from familiar practices there should be independent input from the scientific community, organized medicine, industry, the public, and others, in addition to the federal government, to prevent abuse from any sector of society, private or public. Such departures include the use of novel vectors, gene transfer in utero, potential germ line modification, and gene transfer to normal volunteers.

If and when gene replacement with normal DNA becomes a practical reality for the treatment of human disorders, the following factors should be considered:
(1) If procedures are performed in a research setting, reference should be made to the Council's guidelines on clinical investigation.
(2) If procedures are performed in a non-research setting, adherence to usual and customary standards of medical practice and professional responsibility would be required.

(3) Full discussion of the proposed procedure with the patient would be required. The consent of the patient or the patient's legal representative should be informed, voluntary and written.

(4) There must be no hazardous or other unwanted virus on the viral DNA containing the replacement or corrective gene.

(5) The inserted DNA must function under normal control within the recipient cell to prevent metabolic damage that could damage tissue and the patient.

(6) The effectiveness of the gene therapy should be evaluated as well as possible. This will include determination of the natural history of the disease and follow-up examination of subsequent generations.

(7) Such procedures should be undertaken in the future only after careful evaluation of the availability and effectiveness of other possible therapy. If simpler and safer treatment is available, it should be pursued.

(8) These considerations should be reviewed, as appropriate, as procedures and scientific information are developed in the future. (I, V, VII)

Issued March 1980.

Updated June 1996.

2.132 Genetic Testing by Employers

As a result of the human genome project, physicians will be able to identify a greater number of genetic risks of disease. Among the potential uses of the tests that detect these risks will be screening of potential workers by employers. Employers may want to exclude workers with certain genetic risks from the workplace because these workers may become disabled prematurely, impose higher health care costs, or pose a risk to public safety. In addition, exposure to certain substances in the workplace may increase the likelihood that a disease will develop in the worker with a genetic risk for the disease.

(1) It would generally be inappropriate to exclude workers with genetic risks of disease from the workplace because of their risk. Genetic tests alone do not have sufficient predictive value to be relied upon as a basis for excluding workers. Consequently, use of the tests would result in unfair discrimination against individuals who have positive test results. In addition, there are other ways for employers to serve their legitimate interests. Tests of a worker's actual capacity to meet the demands of the job can be used to ensure future employability and protect the public's safety. Routine monitoring of a worker's exposure can be used to protect workers who have a genetic susceptibility to injury from a substance in the workplace. In addition, employees should be advised of the risks of injury to which they are being exposed.

(2) There may be a role for genetic testing in the exclusion from the workplace of workers who have a genetic susceptibility to injury. At a minimum, several conditions would have to be met:

(a) The disease develops so rapidly that serious and irreversible injury would occur before monitoring of either the worker's exposure to the toxic substance or the worker's health status could be effective in preventing the harm.

(b) The genetic testing is highly accurate, with sufficient sensitivity and specificity to minimize the risk of false negative and false positive test results.

(c) Empirical data demonstrate that the genetic abnormality results in an unusually elevated susceptibility to occupational injury.

(d) It would require undue cost to protect susceptible employees by lowering the level of the toxic substance in the workplace. The costs of lowering the level of the substance must be extraordinary relative to the employer's other costs of making the product for which the toxic substance is used. Since genetic testing with exclusion of susceptible employees is the alternative to cleaning up the workplace, the cost of lowering the level of the substance must also be extraordinary relative to the costs of using genetic testing.

(e) Testing must not be performed without the informed consent of the employee or applicant for employment. (IV)

Issued June 1991 based on the report "Genetic Testing by Employers," adopted June 1991 (JAMA. 1991; 266: 1827-1830).

2.135 Insurance Companies and Genetic Information

Physicians should not participate in genetic testing by health insurance companies to predict a person's predisposition for disease. As a corollary, it may be necessary for physicians to maintain separate files for genetic testing results to ensure that the results are not sent to health insurance companies when requests for copies of patient medical records are fulfilled. Physicians who withhold testing results should inform insurance companies that, when medical records are sent, genetic testing results are not included. This disclosure should occur with all patients, not just those who have undergone genetic testing. (IV)

Issued June 1994 based on the report "Physician Participation in Genetic Testing by Health Insurance Companies," adopted June 1993.

Updated June 1996.

2.137 Ethical Issues in Carrier Screening of Genetic Disorders

All carrier testing must be voluntary, and informed consent from screened individuals is required. Confidentiality of results is to be maintained. Results of testing should not be disclosed to third parties without the explicit informed consent of the screened individual. Patients should be informed as to potential uses for the genetic information by third parties, and whether other ways of obtaining the information are available when appropriate.

Carrier testing should be available uniformly among the at-risk population being screened. One legitimate exception to this principle is the limitation of carrier testing to individuals of childbearing age. In pursuit of uniform access, physicians should not limit testing only to patients specifically requesting testing. If testing is offered to some patients, it should be offered to all patients within the same risk category.

The direction of future genetic screening tests should be determined by well thought out and well-coordinated social policy. Third parties, including insurance companies or employers, should not be permitted to discriminate against carriers of genetic disorders through policies which have the ultimate effect of influencing decisions about testing and reproduction. (IV, V)

Issued June 1994 based on the report "Ethical Issues in Carrier Screening for Cystic Fibrosis and Other Genetic Disorders," adopted June 1991.

2.138 Genetic Testing of Children

Genetic testing of children implicates important concerns about individual autonomy and the interest of the patients. Before testing of children can be performed, there must be some potential benefit from the testing that can reasonably be viewed as outweighing the disadvantages of testing, particularly the harm from abrogating the children's future choice in knowing their genetic status. When there is such a potential benefit, parents should decide whether their children will undergo testing. If parents unreasonably request or refuse testing of their child, physician should take steps to change or, if necessary, use legal means to override the parents' choice. Applying these principles to specific circumstances yields the following conclusions:

(1) When a child is a risk for a genetic condition for which preventive or other therapeutic measures are available, genetic testing should be offered or, in some cases, required.

(2) When a child is a risk for a genetic condition with pediatric onset for which preventive or other therapeutic measures are not available, parents generally should have discretion to decide about genetic testing.

(3) When a child is at risk for a genetic condition with adult onset for which preventive or other therapeutic measures are not available, genetic testing of children generally should not be undertaken. Families should still be informed of the existence of tests and given the opportunity to discuss the reasons why the tests are generally not offered for children.

(4) Genetic testing for carrier status should be deferred until either the child reaches maturity, the child needs to make reproductive decisions or, in the case of children too immature to make their own reproductive decisions, reproductive decisions need to be made for the child.

(5) Genetic testing of children for the benefit of a family member should not be performed unless the testing is necessary to prevent substantial harm to the family member.

When a child's genetic status is determined incidentally, the information should be retained by the physician and entered into the patient record. Discussion of the existence of this finding should then be taken up when the child reaches maturity or needs to make reproductive decisions, so that the individual can decide whether to request disclosure of the information. It is important that physicians be consistent in disclosing both positive and negative results in the same way since if physicians raise the existence of the testing results only when the results are positive, individuals will know what the results must be. This information should not be disclosed to third parties. Genetic information should be maintained in a separate portion of the medical record to prevent mistaken disclosure.

When a child is being considered for adoption, the guidelines for genetic testing should be the same as for other children. (IV)

Issued June 1996 based on the report "Testing Children for Genetic Status," adopted June 1995.

2.139 Multiplex Genetic Testing

Multiplex testing—where tests are offered for several different medical conditions in a single session—presents a series of challenges to adequate communication between the patient and the physician. It increases the total number of marginally indicated or non-indicated tests, thereby bolstering the rate of false results. These results may lead to psychological stress and misinformed life-altering decisions, and may also impact the ability of a physician to obtain informed consent. Multiplex testing and its resultant information may also have widespread societal implications that include discriminatory practices against not only individuals but specific ethnic groups that have been designated "at risk" populations.

Before such tests reach health care providers, clinics, and drugstores, the ethical and social implications of these tests must be well-understood, and careful restrictions and regulations must be established. The following guidelines are offered on the future possibilities of multiplex genetic testing:
(1) Physicians should not routinely order tests for multiple genetic conditions.
(2) Tests for more than one genetic condition should be ordered only when clinically relevant and after the patient has had full counseling and has given informed consent for each test.
(3) Efforts should be made to educate clinicians and society about the uncertainty surrounding genetic testing. (IV, V)

Issued June 1998 based on the report "Multiplex Genetic Testing," adopted December 1996.

2.14 In Vitro Fertilization

The technique of in vitro fertilization and embryo transplantation enables certain couples previously incapable of conception to bear a child. It is also useful in the field of research directed toward an understanding of how genetic defects arise and are transmitted and how they might be prevented or treated. Because of serious ethical and moral concerns, however, any fertilized egg that has the potential for human life and that will be implanted in the uterus of a woman should not be subjected to laboratory research.

All fertilized ova not utilized for implantation and that are maintained for research purposes shall be handled with the strictest adherence to the Principles of Medical Ethics, to the guidelines for research and medical practice expressed in the Council's opinion on fetal research, and to the highest standards of medical practice. (I, V, VII)

Issued June 1983.

2.141 Frozen Pre-embryos

The practice of freezing extra pre-embryos harvested during the in vitro fertilization process (IVF) has enhanced the ability of infertile couples to preserve embryos for future implantation. This practice has also posed a number of ethical and legal dilemmas, including questions regarding decision making authority over the pre-embryos and appropriate uses of pre-embryos.

This country's cultural and legal traditions indicate that the logical persons to exercise control over a frozen pre-embryo are the woman and man who provided the gametes (the ovum and sperm). The gamete providers have a fundamental interest at stake, their potential for procreation. In addition, the gamete providers are the parties most concerned with the interests of a frozen pre-embryo and most likely to protect those interests.

Gamete providers should be able to use the pre-embryos themselves or donate them for use by other parties, but not sell them. In addition, research on pre-embryos should be permitted as long as the pre-embryos are not destined for transfer to a woman for implantation and as long as the research is conducted in accordance with the Council's guidelines on fetal research. Frozen pre-embryos may also be allowed to thaw and deteriorate.

The gamete providers should have an equal say in the use of their pre-embryos and, therefore, the pre-embryos should not be available for use by either provider or changed from their frozen state without the consent of both providers. The man and woman each has contributed half of the pre-embryo's genetic code. In addition, whether a person chooses to become a parent and assume all of the accompanying obligations is a particularly personal and fundamental decision. Even if the individual could be absolved of any parental obligations, he or she may have a strong desire not to have offspring. The absence of a legal duty does not eliminate the moral duty many would feel toward any genetic offspring.

Advance agreements are recommended for deciding the disposition of frozen pre-embryos in the event of divorce or other changes in circumstances. Advance agreements can help ensure that the gamete providers undergo IVF and pre-embryo freezing after a full contemplation of the consequences but should not be mandatory. (I, III, IV, V)

Issued March 1992 based on the report "Frozen Pre-Embryos," adopted December 1989 (JAMA. 1990; 263: 2484-2487).

Updated June 1994.

2.145 Pre-embryo Splitting

The technique of splitting in vitro fertilized pre-embryos may result in multiple genetically identical siblings.

The procedure of pre-embryo splitting should be available so long as both gamete providers agree. This procedure may greatly increase the chances of conception for an infertile couple or for a couple whose future reproductive capacity will likely be diminished. Pre-embryo splitting also can reduce the number of invasive procedures necessary for egg retrieval and the necessity for hormonal stimulants to generate multiple eggs. The use and disposition of any pre-embryos that are frozen for future use should be consistent with the Council's opinion on frozen pre-embryos. (Opinion 2.141)

The use of frozen pre-embryo identical siblings many years after one child has been born raises new ethical issues. Couples might wait until they can discover the mental and physical characteristics of a child before transferring a genetically identical sibling for implantation, they might sell their frozen pre-embryos based upon the outcome of a genetically identical child, or they might decide to transplant a genetically identical sibling based on the need to harvest the child's tissue.

The Council does not find that these considerations are sufficient to prohibit pre-embryo splitting for the following reasons:

(1) It would take many years to determine the outcome of a child and most families want to complete their childbearing within a shorter time.

(2) The sale of pre-embryos can and should be prohibited.

(3) The small number of couples who might bear identical siblings solely for purposes of harvesting their tissue does not outweigh the benefits which might be derived from pre-embryo splitting. Additionally, it is not evident that a sibling would have negative psychological or emotional consequences from having acted as an organ or tissue donor. Indeed, the child may derive psychological benefits from having saved the life of a sibling.

To the extent possible, discussion of these issues should be had with gamete providers prior to pre-embryo splitting and freezing so as to inform the prospective parents of possible future ethical dilemmas. (I, III, IV, V)

Issued June 1994.

2.147 Human Cloning

"Somatic cell nuclear transfer" is the process in which the nucleus of a somatic cell of an organism is transferred into an enucleated oocyte. "Human cloning" is the application of somatic nuclear transfer technology to the creation of a human being that shares all of its nuclear genes with the person donating the implanted nucleus.

In order to clarify the many existing misconceptions about human cloning, physicians should help educate the public about the intrinsic limits of human cloning as well as the current ethical and legal protections that would prevent abuses of human cloning. These include the following: (1) using human cloning as an approach to terminal illness or mortality is a concept based on the mistaken notion that one's genotype largely determines one's individuality. A clone-child created via human cloning would not be identical to his or her clone-parent. (2) Current ethical and legal standards hold that under no circumstances should human cloning occur without an individual's permission. (3) Current ethical and legal standards hold that a human clone would be entitled to the same rights, freedoms, and protections as every other individual in society. The fact that a human clone's nuclear genes would derive from a single individual rather than two parents would not change his or her moral standing.

Physicians have an ethical obligation to consider the harms and benefits of new medical procedures and technologies. Physicians should not participate in human cloning at this time because further investigation and discussion regarding the harms and benefits of human cloning is required. Concerns include: (1) unknown physical harms introduced by cloning. Somatic cell nuclear transfer has not yet been refined and its long-term safety has not yet been proven. The risk of producing individuals with genetic anomalies gives rise to an obligation to seek better understanding of—and potential medical therapies for—the unforeseen medical consequences that could stem from human cloning. (2) Psychosocial harms introduced by cloning, including violations of privacy and autonomy. Human cloning risks limiting, at least psychologically, the seemingly unlimited potential of new human beings and thus creating enormous pressures on the clone-child to live up to expectations based on the life of the clone-parent. (3) The impact of human cloning on familial and societal relations. The family unit may be altered with the introduction of cloning, and more thought is required on a societal level regarding how to construct familial relations. (4) Potential effects on the gene pool. Like other interventions that can change individuals' reproductive patterns and the resulting genetic characteristics of a population, human cloning has the potential to be used in a eugenic or discriminatory fashion—practices that are incompatible with the ethical norms of medical practice. Moreover, human cloning could alter irreversibly the gene pool and exacerbate genetic problems that arise from deleterious genetic mutations, resulting in harms to future generations.

Two potentially realistic and possibly appropriate medical uses of human cloning are for assisting individuals or couples to reproduce and for the generation of tissues when the donor is not harmed or sacrificed. Given the unresolved issues regarding cloning identified above, the medical profession should not undertake human cloning at this time and pursue alternative approaches that raise fewer ethical concerns.

Because cloning technology is not limited to the United States, physicians should help establish international guidelines governing human cloning. (V)

Issued December 1999 based on the report "The Ethics of Human Cloning," adopted June 1999.

2.15 Financial Incentives for Organ Donation

The voluntary donation of organs in appropriate circumstances is to be encouraged. However, it is not ethical to participate in a procedure to enable a living donor to receive payment, other than for the reimbursement of expenses necessarily incurred in connection with removal, for any of the donor's non-renewable organs.

Procedures involving financial incentives for cadaveric organ donors should have adequate safeguards to ensure that the health of donors and recipients is in no way jeopardized, and that the quality of the organ supply is not degraded. Incentives should be limited to future contracts offered to prospective donors. By entering into a future contract, an adult would agree while still competent to donate his or her organs after death. In return, the donor's family or estate would receive some financial remuneration after the organs have been retrieved and judged medically suitable for transplantation. Several other conditions would apply:

(1) Only the potential donor, and not the donor's family or other third party, may be given the option of accepting financial incentives for cadaveric organ donation. In addition, the potential donor must be a competent adult when the decision to donate is made, and the donor must not have committed suicide.

(2) Any incentive should be of moderate value and should be the lowest amount that can reasonably be expected to encourage organ donation. By designating a state agency to administer the incentive, full control over the level of incentive can be maintained.

(3) Payment should occur only after the organs have been retrieved and judged medically suitable for transplantation. Suitability should continue to be determined in accordance with the procedures of the Organ Procurement and Transplantation Network.

(4) Incentives should play no part in the allocation of donated organs among potential transplant recipients. The distribution of organs for transplantation should continue to be governed only by ethically appropriate criteria relating to medical need. (I, III, V)

Issued June 1984.

Updated June 1994 based on the report "Financial Incentives for Organ Procurement: Ethical Aspects of Future Contracts for Cadaveric Donors," adopted December 1993.

2.155 Mandated Choice and Presumed Consent for Cadaveric Organ Donation

A system of mandated choice for organ donation, in which individuals are required to express their preferences regarding organ donation when renewing their drivers' licenses or performing some other state-mandated task, is an ethically appropriate strategy for encouraging donation and should be pursued. To be effective, information on the importance of organ donation and the success of organ transplantation should be provided when the donation decision is made.

A system of presumed consent for organ donation, in which individuals are assumed to consent to be organ donors after death unless they indicate their refusal to consent, raises serious ethical concerns. For presumed consent to be ethically acceptable, effective mechanisms for documenting and honoring refusals to donate must be in place. In addition, when there is no documented refusal by the individual decedent, the family of the decedent would have to be contacted to verify that they do not know of any objections to donation by the decedent while living. (I, III, V)

Issued June 1994 based on the report "Strategies for Cadaveric Organ Procurement: Mandated Choice and Presumed Consent," adopted December 1993.

2.157 Organ Procurement Following Cardiac Death

Given the increasing need for donor organs, protocols for procurement following cardiac death have been developed. In some instances, patients or their surrogate decision makers request withdrawal of life support and choose to serve as organ donors. In these cases, the organs can be preserved best by discontinuation of life support in the operating room so that organs can be removed two minutes following cardiac death. In other scenarios, patients who suffer unexpected cardiac death may be cannulated and perfused with cold preserving fluid (in situ preservation) to maintain organs. Both of these methods may be ethically permissible, with attention to certain safeguards.

(1) When securing consent for life support withdrawal and organ retrieval, the health care team must be certain that consent is voluntary. This is particularly true where surrogate decisions about life-sustaining treatment may be influenced by the prospect of organ donation. If there is any reason to suspect undue influence, a full ethics consultation should be required.

(2) In all instances, it is critical that there be no conflict of interest in the health care team. Those health care professionals providing care at the end of life must be separated from providers participating in the transplant team.

(3) Further pilot programs should assess the success and acceptability of organ removal following withdrawal of life-sustaining treatment.

(4) In cases of in situ preservation of cadaveric organs, the prior consent of the decedent or the consent of the decedent's surrogate decision maker makes perfusion ethically permissible. Perfusion without either prior specific consent to perfusion or general consent to organ donation violates requirements for informed consent for medical procedures and should not be permitted.

(5) The recipients of such procured organs should be informed of the source of the organs as well as any potential defects in the quality of the organs, so that they may decide with their physicians whether to accept the organs or wait for more suitable ones.

(6) Clear clinical criteria should be developed to ensure that only appropriate candidates, whose organs are reasonably likely to be suitable for transplantation, are considered eligible to donate organs under these protocols.
(I, III, V)

Issued June 1996 based on the reports "Ethical Issues in the Procurement of Organs Following Cardiac Death: The Pittsburgh Protocol," and "Ethical Issues in Organ Procurement Following Cardiac Death: In Situ Preservation of Cadaveric Organs," adopted December 1994.

2.16 Organ Transplantation Guidelines

The following statement is offered for guidance of physicians as they seek to maintain the highest level of ethical conduct in the transplanting of human organs.

(1) In all professional relationships between a physician and a patient, the physician's primary concern must be the health of the patient. The physician owes the patient primary allegiance. This concern and allegiance must be preserved in all medical procedures, including those which involve the transplantation of an organ from one person to another where both donor and recipient are patients. Care must, therefore, be taken to protect the rights of both the donor and the recipient, and no physician may

assume a responsibility in organ transplantation unless the rights of both donor and recipient are equally protected. A prospective organ transplant offers no justification for a relaxation of the usual standard of medical care for the potential donor.

(2) When a vital, single organ is to be transplanted, the death of the donor shall have been determined by at least one physician other than the recipient's physician. Death shall be determined by the clinical judgment of the physician, who should rely on currently accepted and available scientific tests.

(3) Full discussion of the proposed procedure with the donor and the recipient or their responsible relatives or representatives is mandatory. The physician should ensure that consent to the procedure is fully informed and voluntary, in accordance with the Council's guidelines on informed consent. The physician's interest in advancing scientific knowledge must always be secondary to his or her concern for the patient.

(4) Transplant procedures of body organs should be undertaken (a) only by physicians who possess special medical knowledge and technical competence developed through special training, study, and laboratory experience and practice, and (b) in medical institutions with facilities adequate to protect the health and well-being of the parties to the procedure.

(5) Recipients of organs for transplantation should be determined in accordance with the Council's guidelines on the allocation of limited medical resources.

(6) Organs should be considered a national, rather than a local or regional, resource. Geographical priorities in the allocation of organs should be prohibited except when transportation of organs would threaten their suitability for transplantation.

(7) Patients should not be placed on the waiting lists of multiple local transplant centers, but rather on a single waiting list for each type of organ. (I, III, V)

Issued prior to April 1977.

Updated June 1994 based on the report "Ethical Considerations in the Allocation of Organs and Other Scarce Medical Resources Among Patients," adopted June 1993.

2.161 Medical Applications of Fetal Tissue Transplantation

The principal ethical concern in the use of human fetal tissue for transplantation is the degree to which the decision to have an abortion might be influenced by the decision to donate the fetal tissue. In the application of fetal tissue transplantation the following safeguards should apply: (1) The Council on Ethical and Judicial Affairs' guidelines on clinical investigation and organ transplantation are followed, as they pertain to the recipient of the fetal tissue transplant (see Opinion 2.07, Clinical Investigation, and Opinion 2.16, Organ Transplantation Guidelines); (2) a final decision regarding abortion is made before initiating a discussion of the transplantation use of fetal tissue; (3) decisions regarding the technique used to induce abortion, as well as the timing of the abortion in relation to the gestational age of the fetus, are based on concern for the safety of the pregnant woman; (4) fetal tissue is not provided in exchange for financial remuneration above that which is necessary to cover reasonable expenses; (5) the recipient of the tissue is not designated by the donor; (6) health care personnel involved in the termination of a particular pregnancy do not participate in or receive any benefit from the transplantation of tissue from the abortus of the same pregnancy; and (7) informed consent on behalf of both the donor and the recipient is obtained in accordance with applicable law. (I, IV, V)

Issued March 1992 based on the report "Medical Applications of Fetal Tissue Transplantation," adopted June 1989 (JAMA. 1990; 263: 565-570).

Updated June 1996.

2.162   Anencephalic Neonates as Organ Donors

Anencephaly is a congenital absence of major portion of the brain, skull, and scalp. Anencephalic neonates are thought to be unique from other brain-damaged beings because of a lack of past consciousness with no potential for future consciousness.

Physicians may provide anencephalic neonates with ventilator assistance and other medical therapies that are necessary to sustain organ perfusion and viability until such time as a determination of death can be made in accordance with accepted medical standards, relevant law and regional organ procurement organization policy. Retrieval and transplantation of the organs of anencephalic infants are ethically permissible only after such determination of death is made, and only in accordance with the Council's guidelines for transplantation. (I, III, V)

Issued March 1992 based on the report "Anencephalic Infants as Organ Donors," adopted December 1988.

Updated June 1994; updated December 1994 based on the report "The Use of Anencephalic Neonates as Organ Donors," adopted December 1994; and updated June 1996 based on the report "Anencephalic Infants as Organ Donors—Reconsideration," adopted December 1995.

2.165   Fetal Umbilical Cord Blood

Human umbilical cord blood has been identified as a viable source of hematopoietic stem cells that can be used as an alternative to bone marrow for transplantation. It is obtained by clamping the umbilical cord immediately after delivery.

The use of umbilical cord blood raises two main ethical problems. First, the exact timing of the clamping has a significant impact on the neonate. Studies indicate that early clamping may cause an abrupt surge in arterial pressure, resulting in intraventricular hemorrhage (particularly in premature infants). Second, there is a risk that the infant donor will develop a need for his or her own cord blood later in life. If that child was a donor and this later need arises, he or she might be without blood, when he or she could have had his or her own blood stored.

To avoid health risks, normal clamping protocol should be followed and not altered in such a way that might endanger the infant. Additionally, parents of the infant must be fully informed of the risks of the donation and written consent should be obtained from them.

The second concern, that the child may need the blood later in life, is more complex. The possibility that an infant donor would be in need of his or her own umbilical cord blood is highly speculative. There are a number of reasons why the infant may not need the blood later. The diseases that are treated by bone marrow transplantation are not common, and there may be other treatment alternatives available, particularly in the future when the illness would occur. Additionally, the demand for fetal umbilical cord blood will increase as it becomes medically certain that the blood may be used in persons unrelated to the donor. This situation will reduce the need to store a particular infant's blood since umbilical cord blood from other donors would be available. If the blood is sufficient for use in unrelated individuals, then the donor may obtain the cord blood from another donor later in life, making the need to store his or her own blood unnecessary. These original donors, however, should be given priority in receipt of such blood if they need a donation later in life.

For all of these reasons, it would generally not be unethical to use the cord blood. However, if the child-donor is known to be at risk for an illness that is treated by bone marrow donation, the child should not be used as a donor, and his or her blood should be stored for future use. (I, V)

Issued June 1994.

Updated June 1996.

2.167 The Use of Minors as Organ and Tissue Donors

Minors need not be prohibited from acting as sources of organs, but their participation should be limited. Different procedures pose different degrees of risk and do not all require the same restrictions. In general, minors should not be permitted to serve as a source when there is a very serious risk of complications (e.g., partial liver or lung donation, which involve a substantial risk of serious immediate or long-term morbidity). If the safeguards in the remainder of this opinion are followed, minors may be permitted to serve as a source when the risks are low (e.g., blood or skin donation, in which the donated tissue can regenerate and spinal or general anesthesia is not required), moderate (e.g., bone marrow donation, in which the donated tissue can regenerate but brief general or spinal anesthesia is required) or serious (e.g., kidney donation, which involve more extensive anesthesia and major invasive surgery).

If a child is capable of making his or her own medical treatment decisions, he or she should be considered capable of deciding whether to be an organ or tissue donor. However, physicians should not perform organ retrievals of serious risk without first obtaining court authorization. Courts should confirm that the mature minor is acting voluntarily and without coercion.

If a child is not capable of making his or her own medical decisions, all transplantations should have parental approval, and those which pose a serious risk should receive court authorization. In the court authorization process, the evaluation of a child psychiatrist or psychologist must be sought and a guardian ad litem should be assigned to the potential minor donor in order to fully represent the minor's interests.

When deciding on behalf of immature children, parents and courts should ensure that transplantation presents a "clear benefit" to the minor source, which entails meeting the following requirements:

(1) Ideally the minor should be the only possible source. All other available sources of organs, both donor pools and competent adult family members, must be medically inappropriate or significantly inferior. An unwilling potential donor does not qualify him/her as medically inappropriate.

(2) For transplantations of moderate or serious risk, the transplantation must be necessary with some degree of medical certainty to provide a substantial benefit; that is, it both prevents an extremely poor quality of life and ensures a good quality of life for the recipient. A transplant should not be allowed if it merely increases the comfort of the recipient. If a transplant is not presently considered to provide a substantial benefit but is expected to do so within a period of time, the transplant need not be delayed until it meets this criterion, especially if the delay would significantly decrease the benefits derived from the transplant by the recipient.

(3) The organ or tissue transplant must have a reasonable probability of success in order for transplantation to be allowed. What constitutes a reasonable chance of success should be based on medical judgments about the physical condition of the recipient and the likelihood that the transplant will not be rejected, futile, or produce benefits which are very transient. Children should not be used for transplants that are considered experimental or non-standard.

(4) Generally, minors should be allowed to serve as a source only to close family members.

(5) Psychological or emotional benefits to the potential source may be considered, though evidence of future benefit to the minor source should be clear and convincing. Possible benefits to a child include continued emotional bonds between the minor and the recipient, increased self-esteem, and prevention of adverse reaction to death of a sibling. Whether a child will capture these benefits depends upon the child's specific circumstances. A minor's assent or dissent to a procedure is an important piece of evidence that demonstrates whether the transplant will offer psychological benefits to the source. Dissent from incompetent minors should be powerful evidence that the donation will not provide a clear benefit, but may not present an absolute bar. Every effort should be made to identify and address the child's concerns in this case.

(6) It is essential to ensure that the potential source does not have any underlying conditions that create an undue individual risk. (I, V)

Issued June 1994 based on the report "The Use of Minors as Organ and Tissue Donors," adopted December 1993.

2.17 Quality of Life

In the making of decisions for the treatment of seriously disabled newborns or of other persons who are severely disabled by injury or illness, the primary consideration should be what is best for the individual patient and not the avoidance of a burden to the family or to society. Quality of life, as defined by the patient's interests and values, is a factor to be considered in determining what is best for the individual. It is permissible to consider quality of life when deciding about life-sustaining treatment in accordance with Opinions 2.20, 2.215, and 2.22. (I, III, IV)

Issued March 1981.

Updated June 1994.

2.18 Surrogate Mothers

"Surrogate" motherhood involves the artificial insemination of a woman who agrees, usually in return for payment, to give the resulting child to the child's father by surrendering her parental rights. Often, the father's infertile wife becomes the child's adoptive mother. The woman bearing the child is in most cases genetically related to the child, though gestational surrogacy (in which the ovum is provided by the father's infertile wife or other donor) is possible as well.

Ethical, social, and legal problems may arise in surrogacy arrangements. Surrogate motherhood may commodify children and women's reproductive capacities, exploit poor women whose decision to participate may not be wholly voluntary, and improperly discourage or interfere with the formation of a natural maternal-fetal or maternal-child bond. Psychological impairment may occur in a woman who deliberately conceives with the intention of bearing a child which she will give up. In addition, the woman who has contracted to bear the child may decide to have an abortion or to refuse to relinquish her parental rights. Alternatively, if there is a subsequent birth of a disabled child, prospective parents and the birth mother may not want to or will be unable to assume the responsibilities of parenthood.

On the other hand, surrogate motherhood arrangements are often the last hope of prospective parents to have a child that is genetically related to at least one of them. In addition, most surrogacy arrangements are believed by the parties involved to be mutually beneficial, and most are completed without mishap or dispute. In light of the concerns expressed above, however, some safeguards are necessary to protect the welfare of the child and the birth mother. The Council believes that surrogacy contracts, while permissible, should grant the birth mother the right to void the contract within a reasonable period of time after the birth of the child. If the contract is voided, custody of the child should be determined according to the child's best interests.

In gestational surrogacy, in which the surrogate mother has no genetic tie to the fetus, the justification for allowing the surrogate mother to void the contract becomes less clear. Gestational surrogacy contracts should be strictly enforceable (i.e., not voidable by either party). (I, II, IV)

Issued December 1983.

Updated June 1994.

2.19 Unnecessary Services

Physicians should not provide, prescribe, or seek compensation for services that they know are unnecessary. (II, VII)

Issued prior to April 1977.

Updated June 1996.

2.20 Withholding or Withdrawing Life-Sustaining Medical Treatment

The social commitment of the physician is to sustain life and relieve suffering. Where the performance of one duty conflicts with the other, the preferences of the patient should prevail. The principle of patient autonomy requires that physicians respect the decision to forego life-sustaining treatment of a patient who possesses decision-making capacity. Life-sustaining treatment is any treatment that serves to prolong life without reversing the underlying medical condition. Life-sustaining treatment may include, but is not limited to, mechanical ventilation, renal dialysis, chemotherapy, antibiotics, and artificial nutrition and hydration.

There is no ethical distinction between withdrawing and withholding life-sustaining treatment.

A competent, adult patient may, in advance, formulate and provide a valid consent to the withholding or withdrawal of life-support systems in the event that injury or illness renders that individual incompetent to make such a decision. A patient may also appoint a surrogate decision maker in accordance with state law.

If the patient receiving life-sustaining treatment is incompetent, a surrogate decision maker should be identified. Without an advance directive that designates a proxy, the patient's family should become the surrogate decision maker. Family includes persons with whom the patient is closely associated. In the case when there is no person closely associated with the patient, but there are persons who both care about the patient and have sufficient relevant knowledge of the patient, such persons may be appropriate surrogates. Physicians should provide all relevant medical information and explain to surrogate decision makers that decisions regarding withholding or withdrawing life-sustaining treatment should be based on substituted judgment (what the patient would have decided) when there is evidence of the patient's preferences and values. In making a substituted judgment, decision makers may consider the patient's advance directive (if any); the patient's values about life and the way it should be lived; and the patient's attitudes towards sickness, suffering, medical procedures, and death. If there is not adequate evidence of the incompetent patient's preferences and values, the decision should be based on the best interests of the patient (what outcome would most likely promote the patient's well-being).

Though the surrogate's decision for the incompetent patient should almost always be accepted by the physician, there are four situations that may require either institutional or judicial review and/or intervention in the decision-making process: (1) there is no available family member willing to be the patient's surrogate decision maker, (2) there is a dispute among family members and there is no decision maker designated in an advance directive, (3) a health care provider believes that the family's decision is clearly not what the patient would have decided if competent, and (4) a health care provider believes that the decision is not a decision that could reasonably be judged to be in the patient's best interests. When there are disputes among family members or between family and health care providers, the use of ethics committees specifically designed to facilitate sound decision making is recommended before resorting to the courts.

When a permanently unconscious patient was never competent or had not left any evidence of previous preferences or values, since there is no objective way to ascertain the best interests of the patient, the surrogate's decision should not be challenged as long as the decision is based on the decision maker's true concern for what would be best for the patient.

Physicians have an obligation to relieve pain and suffering and to promote the dignity and autonomy of dying patients in their care. This includes providing effective palliative treatment even though it may foreseeably hasten death.

Even if the patient is not terminally ill or permanently unconscious, it is not unethical to discontinue all means of life-sustaining medical treatment in accordance with a proper substituted judgment or best interests analysis. (I, III, IV, V)

Issued December 1984 as Opinion 2.18, Withholding or Withdrawing Life-Prolonging Medical Treatment, and Opinion 2.19, Withholding or Withdrawing Life-Prolonging Medical Treatment—Patients' Preferences. In 1989, these Opinions were renumbered 2.20 and 2.21, respectively.

Updated June 1994 based on the reports "Decisions Near the End of Life" and "Decisions to Forego Life-Sustaining Treatment for Incompetent Patients," both adopted June 1991 (JAMA. 1992; 267: 2229-2233), and updated June 1996.

[In March 1981, the Council on Ethical and Judicial Affairs issued Opinion 2.11, Terminal Illness. The Opinion was renumbered 2.15 in 1984 and was deleted in 1986.]

2.21   The previous Opinion 2.21, **Withholding or Withdrawing Life-Prolonging Medical Treatment—Patients' Preferences**, was deleted in 1994 and combined with the current Opinion 2.20.

2.21 Euthanasia

Euthanasia is the administration of a lethal agent by another person to a patient for the purpose of relieving the patient's intolerable and incurable suffering.

It is understandable, though tragic, that some patients in extreme duress — such as those suffering from a terminal, painful, debilitating illness — may come to decide that death is preferable to life. However, permitting physicians to engage in euthanasia would ultimately cause more harm than good. Euthanasia is fundamentally incompatible with the physician's role as healer, would be difficult or impossible to control, and would pose serious societal risks.

The involvement of physicians in euthanasia heightens the significance of its ethical prohibition. The physician who performs euthanasia assumes unique responsibility for the act of ending the patient's life. Euthanasia could also readily be extended to incompetent patients and other vulnerable populations.

Instead of engaging in euthanasia, physicians must aggressively respond to the needs of patients at the end of life. Patients should not be abandoned once it is determined that cure is impossible. Patients near the end of life must continue to receive emotional support, comfort care, adequate pain control, respect for patient autonomy, and good communication. (I, IV)

Issued June 1994 based on the report "Decisions Near the End of Life," adopted June 1991 (JAMA. 1992; 267: 2229-2233).

Updated June 1996.

2.211   Physician-Assisted Suicide

Physician-assisted suicide occurs when a physician facilitates a patient's death by providing the necessary means and/or information to enable the patient to perform the life-ending act (e.g., the physician provides sleeping pills and information about the lethal dose, while aware that the patient may commit suicide).

It is understandable, though tragic, that some patients in extreme duress — such as those suffering from a terminal, painful, debilitating illness — may come to decide that death is preferable to life. However, allowing physicians to participate in assisted suicide would cause more harm than good. Physician assisted suicide is fundamentally incompatible with the physician's role as healer, would be difficult or impossible to control, and would pose serious societal risks.

Instead of participating in assisted suicide, physicians must aggressively respond to the needs of patients at the end of life. Patients should not be abandoned once it is determined that cure is impossible. Multidisciplinary interventions should be sought including specialty consultation, hospice care, pastoral support, family counseling and other modalities. Patients near the end of life must continue to receive emotional support, comfort care, adequate pain control, respect for patient autonomy, and good communication. (I, IV)

Issued 1994 based on the reports "Decisions Near the End of Life," adopted June 1991 and "Physician-Assisted Suicide," adopted December 1993 (JAMA. 1992; 267: 2229-2233).

Updated June 1996.

2.215   Treatment Decisions for Seriously Ill Newborns

The primary consideration for decisions regarding life-sustaining treatment for seriously ill newborns should be what is best for the newborn. Factors that should be weighed are: (1) the chance that therapy will succeed, (2) the risks involved with treatment and nontreatment, (3) the degree to which the therapy, if successful, will extend life, (4) the pain and discomfort associated with the therapy, and (5) the anticipated quality of life for the newborn with and without treatment.

Care must be taken to evaluate the newborn's expected quality of life from the child's perspective. Life-sustaining treatment may be withheld or withdrawn from a newborn when the pain and suffering expected to be endured by the child will overwhelm any potential for joy during his or her life. When an infant suffers extreme neurological damage, and is consequently not capable of experiencing either suffering or joy, a decision may be made to withhold or withdraw life-sustaining treatment. When life-sustaining treatment is withheld or withdrawn, comfort care must not be discontinued.

When an infant's prognosis is largely uncertain, as is often the case with extremely premature newborns, all life-sustaining and life-enhancing treatment should be initiated. Decisions about life-sustaining treatment should be made once the prognosis becomes more certain. It is not necessary to attain absolute or near absolute prognostic certainty before life-sustaining treatment is withdrawn, since this goal is often unattainable and risks unnecessarily prolonging the infant's suffering.

Physicians must provide full information to parents of seriously ill newborns regarding the nature of treatments, therapeutic options and expected prognosis with and without therapy, so that parents can make informed decisions for their children about life-sustaining treatment. Counseling services and an opportunity to talk with persons who have had to make similar decisions should be available to parents. Ethics committees or infant review committees should also be utilized to facilitate parental decision making. These committees should help mediate resolutions of conflicts that may arise among parents, physicians and others involved in the care of the infant. These committees should also be responsible for referring cases to the appropriate public agencies when it is concluded that the parents' decision is not a decision that could reasonably be judged to be in the best interests of the infant. (I, III, IV, V)

Issued June 1994 based on the report "Treatment Decisions for Seriously Ill Newborns," adopted June 1992.

2.22   Do-Not-Resuscitate Orders

Efforts should be made to resuscitate patients who suffer cardiac or respiratory arrest except when circumstances indicate that cardiopulmonary resuscitation (CPR) would be inappropriate or not in accord with the desires or best interests of the patient.

Patients at risk of cardiac or respiratory failure should be encouraged to express in advance their preferences regarding the use of CPR and this should be documented in the patient's medical record. These discussions should include a description of the procedures encompassed by CPR and, when possible, should occur in an outpatient setting when general treatment preferences are discussed, or as early as possible during hospitalization. The physician has an ethical obligation to honor the resuscitation preferences expressed by the patient. Physicians should not permit their personal value judgments about quality of life to obstruct the implementation of a patient's preferences regarding the use of CPR.

If a patient is incapable of rendering a decision regarding the use of CPR, a decision may be made by a surrogate decision maker, based upon the previously expressed preferences of the patient or, if such preferences are unknown, in accordance with the patient's best interests.

If, in the judgment of the attending physician, it would be inappropriate to pursue CPR, the attending physician may enter a do-not-resuscitate (DNR) order into the patient's record. Resuscitative efforts should be considered inappropriate by the attending physician only if they cannot be expected either to restore cardiac or respiratory function to the patient or to meet established ethical criteria, as defined in the Principles of Medical Ethics and Opinions 2.03 and 2.095. When there is adequate time to do so, the physician must first inform the patient, or the incompetent patient's surrogate, of the content of the DNR order, as well as the basis for its implementation. The physician also should be prepared to discuss appropriate alternatives, such as obtaining a second opinion (e.g., consulting a bioethics committee) or arranging for transfer of care to another physician.

DNR orders, as well as the basis for their implementation, should be entered by the attending physician in the patient's medical record.

DNR orders only preclude resuscitative efforts in the event of cardiopulmonary arrest and should not influence other therapeutic interventions that may be appropriate for the patient. (I, IV)

Issued March 1992 based on the report "Guidelines for the Appropriate Use of Do-Not-Resuscitate Orders," adopted December 1990 (JAMA. 1991; 265: 1868-1871).

Updated June 1994.

2.225 Optimal Use of Orders-Not-to-Intervene and Advance Directives

More rigorous efforts in advance care planning are required in order to tailor end-of-life care to the preferences of patients so that they can experience a satisfactory last chapter in their lives. There is need for better availability and tracking of advance directives, and more uniform adoption of form documents that can be honored in all states of the United States. The discouraging evidence of inadequate end-of-life decision-making indicates the necessity of several improvement strategies:

(1) Patients and physicians should make use of advisory as well as statutory documents. Advisory documents aim to accurately represent a patient's wishes and are legally binding under law. Statutory documents give physicians immunity from malpractice for following a patient's wishes. If a form is not available that combines the two, an advisory document should be appended to the state statutory form.

(2) Advisory documents should be based on validated worksheets, thus ensuring reasonable confidence that preferences for end-of-life treatment can be fairly and effectively elicited and recorded, and that they are applicable to medical decisions.

(3) Physicians should directly discuss the patient's preferences with the patient and the patient's proxy. These discussions should be held ahead of time wherever possible. The key steps of structuring a core discussion and of

signing and recording the document in the medical record should not be delegated to a junior member of the health care team.

(4) Central repositories should be established so that completed advisory documents, state statutory documents, identification of a proxy, and identification of the primary physician, can be obtained efficiently in emergency and urgent circumstances as well as routinely.

(5) Health care facilities should honor, and physicians use, a range of orders on the Doctor's Order Sheet to indicate patient wishes regarding avoidable treatments that might otherwise be given on an emergency basis or by a covering physician with less knowledge of the patient's wishes. Treatment avoidance orders might include, along with a Do Not Resuscitate (DNR) order, some of the following: Full Comfort Care Only (FCCO); Do Not Intubate (DNI); Do Not Defibrillate (DND); Do Not Leave Home (DNLH); Do Not Transfer (DNTransfer); No Intravenous Lines (NIL); No Blood Draws (NBD); No Feeding Tube (NFT); No Vital Signs (NVS); and so forth. One common new order, Do Not Treat (DNT), is specifically not included in this list, since it may unintentionally convey the message that no care should be given and the patient may lose the intense attention due to a dying person; FCCO serves the same purpose without the likely misinterpretation. As with DNR orders, these treatment avoidance orders should be revisited periodically to ensure their continued applicability. Active comfort care orders might include Allow Visitors Extended Hours (AVEH); and Inquire About Comfort (IAC) b.i.d. (twice daily). (I, IV)

Issued June 1998 based on the report "Optimal Use of Orders-Not-to-Intervene and Advance Directives," adopted June 1997 (*Pyschology, Public Policy, and Law*. 1998; 4: 668-675).

2.23 HIV Testing

Human Immunodeficiency Virus (HIV) testing is appropriate and should be encouraged for diagnosis and treatment of HIV infection or of medical conditions that may be affected by HIV. Treatment may prolong the lives of those with AIDS and prolong the symptom-free period in those with an asymptomatic HIV infection. Wider testing is imperative to ensure that individuals in need of treatment are identified and treated.

Physicians should ensure that HIV testing is conducted in a way that respects patient autonomy and assures patient confidentiality as much as possible.

The physician should secure the patient's informed consent specific for HIV testing before testing is performed. Because of the need for pretest counseling and the potential consequences of an HIV test on an individual's job, housing, insurability, and social relationships, the consent should be specific for HIV testing. Consent for HIV testing cannot be inferred from a general consent to treatment.

When a health care provider is at risk for HIV infection because of the occurrence of puncture injury or mucosal contact with potentially infected bodily fluids, it is acceptable to test the patient for HIV infection even if the patient refuses consent. When testing without consent is performed in accordance with the law, the patient should be given the customary pretest counseling.

The confidentiality of the results of HIV testing must be maintained as much as possible and the limits of a patient's confidentiality should be known to the patient before consent is given.

Exceptions to confidentiality are appropriate when necessary to protect the public health or when necessary to protect individuals, including health care workers, who are endangered by persons infected with HIV. If a physician knows that a seropositive individual is endangering a third party, the physician should, within the constraints of the law: (1) attempt to persuade the infected patient to cease endangering the third party; (2) if persuasion fails, notify authorities; and (3) if the authorities take no action, notify the endangered third party.

In order to limit the public spread of HIV infection, physicians should encourage voluntary testing of patients at risk for infection.

It is unethical to deny treatment to HIV-infected individuals because they are HIV seropositive or because they are unwilling to undergo HIV testing, except in the instance where knowledge of the patient's HIV status is vital to the appropriate treatment of the patient. When a patient refuses to be tested after being informed of the physician's medical opinion, the physician may transfer the patient to a second physician who is willing to manage the patient's care in accordance with the patient's preferences about testing. (I, IV)

Issued March 1992 based on the report "Ethical Issues Involved in the Growing AIDS Crisis," adopted December 1987 (JAMA. 1988; 259: 1360-1361).

Updated June 1994.

2.30 Information from Unethical Experiments

All proposed experiments using human subjects should undergo proper ethical evaluation by a human studies review board before being undertaken.

Responsibility for revealing that the data are from unethical experiments lies in the hands of authors, peer reviewers, and editors of medical texts that publish results of experimental studies. Each publication should adopt a standard regarding publication of data from unethical experiments.

If data from unethical experiments can be replaced by existing ethically sound data and achieve the same ends, then such must be done. If ethically tainted data that have been validated by rigorous scientific analysis are the only data of that nature available, and such data are necessary in order to save lives, then the utilization of such data by physicians and editors may be appropriate.

Should editors and/or authors decide to publish an experiment or data from an experiment that does not reach standards of contemporary ethical conduct, a disclaimer should be included. Such disclosure would by no means rectify unethical conduct or legitimize the methods of collection of data gathered from unethical experimentation. This disclaimer should: (1) clearly describe the unethical nature of the origin of any material being published; (2) clearly state that publication of the data is needed in order to save human lives; (3) pay respect to the victims; (4) avoid trivializing trauma suffered by the participants; (5) acknowledge the unacceptable nature of the experiments; and (6) endorse higher ethical standards.

Based on both scientific and moral grounds, data obtained from cruel and inhumane experiments, such as data collected from the Nazi experiments and data collected from the Tuskegee Study, should virtually never be published or cited. In the extremely rare case when no other data exist and human lives would certainly be lost without the knowledge obtained from use of such data, publication or citation is permissible. In such a case the disclosure should cite the specific reasons and clearly justify the necessity for citation.

Certain generally accepted historical data may be cited without a disclaimer, though a disclosure of the ethical issues would be valuable and desirable. (II, V, VII)

Issued December 1998 based on the report "Information from Unethical Experiments," adopted June 1998.

3.00 Opinions on Interprofessional Relations

3.01 Nonscientific Practitioners

It is unethical to engage in or to aid and abet in treatment which has no scientific basis and is dangerous, is calculated to deceive the patient by giving false hope, or which may cause the patient to delay in seeking proper care.

Physicians should also be mindful of state laws which prohibit a physician from aiding and abetting an unlicensed person in the practice of medicine, aiding or abetting a person with a limited license in providing services beyond the scope of his or her license, or undertaking the joint medical treatment of patients under the foregoing circumstances.

Physicians are otherwise free to accept or decline to serve anyone who seeks their services, regardless of who has recommended that the individual see the physician. (III, VI)

Issued prior to April 1977.

Updated June 1994 and June 1996.

3.02 Nurses

The primary bond between the practices of medicine and nursing is mutual ethical concern for patients. One of the duties in providing reasonable care is fulfilled by a nurse who carries out the orders of the attending physician. Where orders appear to the nurse to be in error or contrary to customary medical and nursing practice, the physician has an ethical obligation to hear the nurse's concern and explain those orders to the nurse involved. The ethical physician should neither expect nor insist that nurses follow orders contrary to standards of good medical and nursing practice. In emergencies, when prompt action is necessary and the physician is not immediately available, a nurse may be justified in acting contrary to the physician's standing orders for the safety of the patient. Such occurrences should not be considered to be a breakdown in professional relations. (IV, V)

Issued June 1983.

Updated June 1994.

3.03   The previous Opinion 3.03, **Optometry,** was deleted in June 1994.

3.03 Allied Health Professionals

Physicians often practice in concert with allied health professionals such as, but not limited to, optometrists, nurse anesthetists, nurse midwives, and physician assistants in the course of delivering appropriate medical care to their patients. In doing so, physicians should be guided by the following principles:

(1) It is ethical for a physician to work in consultation with or employ allied health professionals, as long as they are appropriately trained and duly licensed to perform the activities being requested.

(2) Physicians have an ethical obligation to the patients for whom they are responsible to insure that medical and surgical conditions are appropriately evaluated and treated.

(3) Physicians may teach in recognized schools for the allied health professionals for the purpose of improving the quality of their education. The scope of teaching may embrace subjects which are within the legitimate scope of the allied health profession and which are designed to prepare students to engage in the practice of the profession within the limits prescribed by law.

(4) It is inappropriate to substitute the services of an allied health professional for those of a physician when the allied health professional is not appropriately trained and duly licensed to provide the medical services being requested. (I, V, VII)

Issued December 1997.

3.04 Referral of Patients

A physician may refer a patient for diagnostic or therapeutic services to another physician, limited practitioner, or any other provider of health care services permitted by law to furnish such services, whenever he or she believes that this may benefit the patient. As in the case of referrals to physician-specialists, referrals to limited practitioners should be based on their individual competence and ability to perform the services needed by the patient. A physician should not so refer a patient unless the physician is confident that the services provided on referral will be performed competently and in accordance with accepted scientific standards and legal requirements. (V, VI)

Issued prior to April 1977.

3.041 Chiropractic

It is ethical for a physician to associate professionally with chiropractors provided that the physician believes that such association is in the best interests of his or her patient. A physician may refer a patient for diagnostic or therapeutic services to a chiropractor permitted by law to furnish such services whenever the physician believes that this may benefit his or her patient. Physicians may also ethically teach in recognized schools of chiropractic. (V, VI)

Issued March 1992.

3.05   The previous Opinion 3.05, **Specialists**, was deleted in June 1994.

3.06 Sports Medicine

Physicians should assist athletes to make informed decisions about their participation in amateur and professional contact sports which entail risks of bodily injury.

The professional responsibility of the physician who serves in a medical capacity at an athletic contest or sporting event is to protect the health and safety of the contestants. The desire of spectators, promoters of the event or even the injured athlete that he or she not be removed from the contest should not be controlling. The physician's judgment should be governed only by medical considerations. (I, VII)

Issued June 1983.

Updated June 1994.

3.07   The previous Opinion 3.07, **Teaching**, was deleted in June 1994.

3.08 Sexual Harassment and Exploitation Between Medical Supervisors and Trainees

Sexual harassment may be defined as sexual advances, requests for sexual favors, and other verbal or physical conduct of a sexual nature when (1) such conduct interferes with an individual's work or academic performance or creates an intimidating, hostile, or offensive work or academic environment or (2) accepting or rejecting such conduct affects or may be perceived to affect employment decisions or academic evaluations concerning the individual. Sexual harassment is unethical.

Sexual relationships between medical supervisors and their medical trainees raise concerns because of inherent inequalities in the status and power that medical supervisors wield in relation to medical trainees and may adversely affect patient care. Sexual relationships between a medical trainee and a supervisor even when consensual are not acceptable regardless of the degree of supervision in any given situation. The supervisory role should be eliminated if the parties involved wish to pursue their relationship. (II, IV, VII)

Issued March 1992 based on the report "Sexual Harassment and Exploitation Between Medical Supervisors and Trainees," adopted June 1989.

Updated June 1994.

4.00 Opinions on Hospital Relations

4.01 Admission Fee

Charging a separate and distinct fee for the incidental, administrative, non-medical service the physician performs in securing the admission of a patient to a hospital is unethical. Physicians should derive their income from medical services rendered, in keeping with the traditions of the American Medical Association. (IV)

Issued prior to April 1977.

Updated June 1994.

4.02 Assessments, Compulsory

It is improper to condition medical staff membership or privileges on compulsory assessments for any purpose. However, self-imposed assessments by vote of the medical staff are acceptable. (IV)

Issued prior to April 1977.

Updated June 1994.

4.03 Billing for Housestaff and Student Services

When a physician assumes responsibility for the services rendered to a patient by a resident or student, the physician may ethically bill the patient for services which were performed under the physician's direct personal observation, direction and supervision. (II)

Issued prior to April 1977.

Updated June 1994.

4.04 Economic Incentives and Levels of Care

The primary obligation of the hospital medical staff is to safeguard the quality of care provided within the institution. The medical staff has the responsibility to perform essential functions on behalf of the hospital in accordance with licensing laws and accreditation requirements. Treatment or hospitalization that is willfully excessive or inadequate constitutes unethical practice. The organized medical staff has an obligation to avoid wasteful practices and unnecessary treatment that may cause the hospital needless expense. In a situation where the economic interests of the hospital are in conflict with patient welfare, patient welfare takes priority. (I, II, IV, V, VI)

Issued June 1986.

4.05 Organized Medical Staff

The organized medical staff performs essential hospital functions even though it may often consist primarily of independent practicing physicians who are not hospital employees. As a practical matter, however, the organized medical staff may enjoy a dual status. In addition to functioning as a division of the hospital, members of the organized medical staff may choose to act as a group for the purpose of communicating and dealing with the governing board and others with respect to matters that concern the interest of the organized medical staff and its members. This is ethical so long as there is no adverse interference with patient care or violation of applicable laws. (IV, VI)

Issued July 1983.

Updated June 1994.

4.06 Physician-Hospital Contractual Relations

There are various financial or contractual arrangements that physicians and hospitals may enter into and find mutually satisfactory. A physician may, for example, be a hospital employee, a hospital-associated medical specialist, or an independent practitioner with staff privileges. The form of the contractual or financial arrangement between physicians and hospitals depends on the facts and circumstances of each situation. A physician may be employed by a hospital for a fixed annual amount, for a certain amount per hour, or pursuant to other similar arrangements that are related to the professional services, skill, education, expertise, or time involved. (VI)

Issued March 1981.

Updated June 1994.

4.07 Staff Privileges

The mutual objective of both the governing board and the medical staff is to improve the quality and efficiency of patient care in the hospital. Decisions regarding hospital privileges should be based upon the training, experience, and demonstrated competence of candidates, taking into consideration the availability of facilities and the overall medical needs of the community, the hospital, and especially patients. Privileges should not be based on numbers of patients admitted to the facility or the economic or insurance status of the patient. Personal friendships, antagonisms, jurisdictional disputes, or fear of competition should not play a role in making these decisions. Physicians who are involved in the granting, denying, or termination of hospital privileges have an ethical responsibility to be guided primarily by concern for the welfare and best interests of patients in discharging this responsibility. (IV, VI, VII)

Issued July 1983.

Updated June 1994.

5.00 Opinions on Confidentiality, Advertising, and Communications Media Relations

5.01 Advertising and Managed Care Organizations

A physician may provide medical services to members of a prepaid medical care plan or to members of a health maintenance organization which seeks members or subscribers through advertising. Physicians practicing in prepaid plans or managed care organizations are subject to the same ethical principles as are other physicians. Advertising which would lead prospective members or subscribers to believe that the services of a named physician who has a reputation for outstanding skill would be routinely available to all members or subscribers, if in fact this is not so, is deceptive. However, the publication by name of the roster of physicians who provide services to members, the type of practice in which each is engaged, biographical and other relevant information is not a deceptive practice. (II, VI)

Issued prior to April 1977.

Updated June 1996.

5.015 Direct-to-Consumer Advertisements of Prescription Drugs

The medical profession needs to take an active role in ensuring that proper advertising guidelines are enforced and that the care patients receive is not compromised as a result of direct-to-consumer advertising. Since the Food and Drug Administration (FDA) has a critical role in determining future directions of direct-to-consumer advertising of prescription drugs, physicians should work to ensure that the FDA remains committed to advertising standards that protect patients' health and safety. Moreover, physicians should encourage and engage in studies regarding the effect of direct-to-consumer adverting on patient health and medical care. Such studies should examine whether direct-to-consumer advertising improves the communication of health information; enhances the patient-physician relationship; and contains accurate and reasonable information on risks, precautions, adverse reactions, and costs.

Physicians must maintain professional standards of informed consent when prescribing. When a patient comes to a physician with a request for a drug he or she has seen advertised, the physician and the patient should engage in a

49

dialogue that would assess and enhance the patient's understanding of the treatment. Although physicians should not be biased against drugs that are advertised, physicians should resist commercially induced pressure to prescribe drugs that may not be indicated. Physicians should deny requests for inappropriate prescriptions and educate patients as to why certain advertised drugs may not be suitable treatment options providing, when available, information on the cost effectiveness of different options.

Physicians must remain vigilant to assure that direct-to-consumer advertising does not promote false expectations. Physicians should be concerned about advertisements that do not enhance consumer education; do not convey a clear, accurate and responsible health education message; do not refer patients to their physicians for more information; do not identify the target population at risk; and fail to discourage consumer self-diagnosis and self-treatment. Physicians may choose to report these concerns directly to the pharmaceutical company that sponsored the advertisement.

To assist the FDA in enforcing existing law and tracking the effects of direct-to-consumer advertising, physicians should, whenever reasonably possible, report to them advertisements that: (1) do not provide a fair and balanced discussion of the use of the drug product for the disease, disorder, or condition; (2) do not clearly explain warnings, precautions, and potential adverse reactions associated with the drug product; (3) do not present summary information in language that can be understood by the consumer; (4) do not comply with applicable FDA rules, regulations, policies and guidelines as provided by the FDA; or (5) do not provide collateral materials to educate both physicians and consumers. (II, III)

Issued June 1999 based on the report "Direct-to-Consumer Advertisements of Prescription Drugs," adopted December 1998 (*Food and Drug Law Journal*. 2000; 55: 119-124).

5.02   Advertising and Publicity

There are no restrictions on advertising by physicians except those that can be specifically justified to protect the public from deceptive practices. A physician may publicize him or herself as a physician through any commercial publicity or other form of public communication (including any newspaper, magazine, telephone directory, radio, television, direct mail, or other advertising) provided that the communication shall not be misleading because of the omission of necessary material information, shall not contain any false or misleading statement, or shall not otherwise operate to deceive.

Because the public can sometimes be deceived by the use of medical terms or illustrations that are difficult to understand, physicians should design the form of communication to communicate the information contained therein to the public in a readily comprehensible manner. Aggressive, high pressure advertising and publicity should be avoided if they create unjustified medical expectations or are accompanied by deceptive claims. The key issue, however, is whether advertising or publicity, regardless of format or content, is true and not materially misleading.

The communication may include: (1) the educational background of the physician; (2) the basis on which fees are determined (including charges for specific services); (3) available credit or other methods of payment; and (4) any other nondeceptive information.

Nothing in this opinion is intended to discourage or to limit advertising and representations which are not false or deceptive within the meaning of Section 5 of the Federal Trade Commission Act. At the same time, however, physicians are advised that certain types of communications have a significant potential for deception and should therefore receive special attention. For example, testimonials of patients as to the physician's skill or the quality of the physician's professional services tend to be deceptive when they do not reflect the results that patients with conditions comparable to the testimoniant's condition generally receive.

Objective claims regarding experience, competence and the quality of physicians and the services they provide may be made only if they are factually supportable. Similarly, generalized statements of satisfaction with a physician's services may be made if they are representative of the experiences of that physician's patients.

Because physicians have an ethical obligation to share medical advances, it is unlikely that a physician will have a truly exclusive or unique skill or remedy. Claims that imply such a skill or remedy therefore can be deceptive. Statements that a physician has an exclusive or unique skill or remedy in a particular geographic area, if true, however, are permissible. Similarly, a statement that a physician has cured or successfully treated a large number of cases involving a particular serious ailment is deceptive if it implies a certainty of result and creates unjustified and misleading expectations in prospective patients.

Consistent with federal regulatory standards which apply to commercial advertising, a physician who is considering the placement of an advertisement or publicity release, whether in print, radio or television, should determine in advance that the communication or message is explicitly and implicitly truthful and not misleading. These standards require the advertiser to have a reasonable basis for claims before they are used in advertising. The reasonable basis must be established by those facts known to the advertiser, and those which a reasonable, prudent advertiser should have discovered. Inclusion of the physician's name in advertising may help to assure that these guidelines are being met. (II)

Issued prior to April 1977.

Updated June 1996

5.025 Physician Advisory or Referral Services by Telecommunication

Telecommunication advisory services, by way of phone, fax or computer, distinct from an existing patient-physician relationship can be a helpful source of medical information for the public. Often, people are not sure where to turn for information of a general medical nature or do not have easy access to other sources of information. Individuals also may be embarrassed about directly bringing up certain questions with their physicians. Although telecommunication advisory services can provide only limited medical services, they can be a useful complement to more comprehensive services, if used properly.

Any telecommunication advisory service should employ certain safeguards to prevent misuse. For example, the physician responding to the call should not make a clinical diagnosis. Diagnosis by telecommunication is done without the benefit of a physician examination or even a face-to-face meeting with the caller. Critical medical data may be unavailable to the physician. Physicians who respond to callers should therefore act within the limitations of telecommunication services and ensure that callers understand the limitations of the services. Under no circumstances should medications be prescribed.

Physicians who respond to the calls should elicit all necessary information from the callers. When callers are charged by the minute, they may try to hurry their calls to limit their costs. As a result, important information may not be disclosed to the physician. Physicians should also ensure that callers do not incur large bills inadvertently or without understanding the billing system.

Physician referral services can also offer important information to the public. Referral services are often provided by medical societies, hospitals and for-profit entities. To ensure that the service bases its recommendation on medically legitimate considerations rather than the likelihood of being paid by the physician, when the service charges physicians a fee to participate, physicians should not pay the service per referral. Also, callers should be told how the list is created. For example, callers should be informed whether the list includes physicians who pay a flat fee to be listed, members of a particular hospital staff or medical society, or physicians who meet some general quality-based criteria.

While these safeguards are described as applying primarily to telephone services, they should be considered equally applicable to any other communication media, such as radio or television in which the physician and patient do not meet face-to-face. (I, IV, VI)

Issued June 1994.

Updated June 1996.

5.03 The previous Opinion 5.03, **Communications Media: Press Relations,** issued prior to April 1977, was deleted in June 1996 and combined with Opinion 5.04.

5.04 Communications Media: Standards of Professional Responsibility

Physicians are ethically and legally required to protect the personal privacy and other legal rights of patients. When information concerning a specific patient is requested by the media, the physician must obtain the consent of the patient or an authorized representative before releasing such information. The physician may release only the authorized information or that which is public knowledge. The patient-physician relationship and its confidential nature must be maintained.

With these considerations in mind, the physician may assist the representatives of the media in every way possible. When the patient or authorized representative consents to the release of information, physicians should cooperate with the press to insure that medical news is available more promptly and more accurately than would be possible without their assistance. Inasmuch as a diagnosis may be made only by a physician and may depend upon X-ray and laboratory studies, no statement regarding diagnosis should be made except by or on behalf of the attending physician. For the same reason, prognosis will be given only by the attending physician or at the attending physician's direction.

Statements regarding the circumstances surrounding shootings, knifings, and poisonings are properly police matters, and questions whether they were accidental should be referred to the appropriate authorities.

Certain news that is part of the public record, such as deaths, may be made available without the consent of the patient or authorized representative. (IV)

Issued prior to 1977.

Updated June 1994 and June 1996.

5.05   Confidentiality

The information disclosed to a physician during the course of the relationship between physician and patient is confidential to the greatest possible degree. The patient should feel free to make a full disclosure of information to the physician in order that the physician may most effectively provide needed services. The patient should be able to make this disclosure with the knowledge that the physician will respect the confidential nature of the communication. The physician should not reveal confidential communications or information without the express consent of the patient, unless required to do so by law.

The obligation to safeguard patient confidences is subject to certain exceptions which are ethically and legally justified because of overriding social considerations. Where a patient threatens to inflict serious bodily harm to another person or to him or herself and there is a reasonable probability that the patient may carry out the threat, the physician should take reasonable precautions for the protection of the intended victim, including notification of law enforcement authorities. Also, communicable diseases, gun shot and knife wounds should be reported as required by applicable statutes or ordinances. (IV)

Issued December 1983.

Updated June 1994.

5.055   Confidential Care for Minors

Physicians who treat minors have an ethical duty to promote the autonomy of minor patients by involving them in the medical decision making process to a degree commensurate with their abilities.

When minors request confidential services, physicians should encourage them to involve their parents. This includes making efforts to obtain the minor's reasons for not involving their parents and correcting misconceptions that may be motivating their objections.

Where the law does not require otherwise, physicians should permit a competent minor to consent to medical care and should not notify parents without the patient's consent. Depending on the seriousness of the decision, competence may be evaluated by physicians for most minors. When necessary, experts in adolescent medicine or child psychological development should be consulted. Use of the courts for competence determinations should be made only as a last resort.

When an immature minor requests contraceptive services, pregnancy-related care (including pregnancy testing, prenatal and postnatal care, and delivery services), or treatment for sexually transmitted disease, drug and alcohol abuse, or mental illness, physicians must recognize that requiring parental involvement may be counterproductive to the health of the patient. Physicians should encourage parental involvement in these situations. However, if the minor continues to object, his or her wishes ordinarily should be respected. If the physician is uncomfortable with providing services without parental involvement, and alternative confidential services are available, the minor may be referred to those services. In cases when the physician believes that without parental involvement and guidance, the minor will face a serious health threat, and there is reason to believe that the parents will be helpful and understanding, disclosing the problem to the parents is ethically justified. When the physician does breach confidentiality to the parents, he or she must discuss the reasons for the breach with the minor prior to the disclosure.

For minors who are mature enough to be unaccompanied by their parents for their examination, confidentiality of information disclosed during an exam, interview, or in counseling should be maintained. Such information may be disclosed to parents when the patient consents to disclosure. Confidentiality may be justifiably breached in situations for which confidentiality for adults may be breached, according to Opinion 5.05. In addition, confidentiality for immature minors may be ethically breached when necessary to enable the parent to make an informed decision about treatment for the minor or when such a breach is necessary to avert serious harm to the minor. (IV)

Issued June 1994 based on the report "Confidential Care for Minors," adopted June 1992.

Updated June 1996.

5.057 Confidentiality of HIV Status on Autopsy Reports

Physicians should maintain the confidentiality of HIV status on autopsy reports to the greatest extent possible.

Physicians who perform autopsies or who have access to autopsy information regarding a patient's HIV status should be familiar with state law governing (1) the reporting of HIV and AIDS to public health authorities; (2) obligations to inform third parties who may be at risk for HIV infection through contact with an HIV-infected decedent; (3) other parties to whom reporting may be required (i.e., funeral directors, health care personnel involved in the care of the patient); and (4) the extent of confidentiality of autopsy records.

HIV status which appears on autopsy records performed under the authority of a hospital are part of the decedent's medical record and should be held confidential. The physician should comply with state laws regarding disclosure to public health authorities and at-risk third parties, and, where such laws are absent, fulfill ethical obligations to notify endangered third parties (e.g., identified sexual or needle-sharing partners). This includes reporting to organ or tissue procurement agencies if any parts of the decedent's body were taken for use in transplantation.

HIV status which appears on autopsy records performed by a medical examiner in the case of suspicious, accidental, or unexplained death should be kept confidential where autopsy records are not accessible to the public. The physician should comply with state laws regarding disclosure to public health authorities and at-risk third parties, and, where such laws are absent, fulfill ethical obligations to notify endangered third parties (e.g., sexual and needle-sharing partners). This includes reporting to organ or tissue procurement agencies if any parts of the decedent's body were taken for use in transplantation.

In cases where autopsies are done under the auspices of the medical examiner's office and state law mandates that the autopsy information be accessible to the public, then physicians should comply with state law. However, in these instances, HIV status should only be recorded when the HIV status of the decedent would be relevant to determining the patient's cause-of-death. In addition, although a patient's HIV status may be learned from public records in some jurisdictions, it is still unethical for a physician to make a public disclosure of an individual patient's HIV status independent of the legal requirements governing the filing or processing of autopsy records. The physician should comply with state laws regarding disclosure to public health authorities and at-risk third parties, and, where such laws are absent, fulfill ethical obligations to notify endangered third parties (e.g., sexual and needle-sharing partners). This includes reporting to organ or tissue procurement agencies if any parts of the decedent's body were taken for use in transplantation. (IV)

Issued June 1994 based on the report "Confidentiality of HIV Status on Autopsy Reports," adopted June 1992 (*Arch Pathol Lab Med.* 1992; 116: 1120-1123).

5.06   Confidentiality: Attorney-Physician Relation

The patient's history, diagnosis, treatment, and prognosis may be discussed with the patient's lawyer with the consent of the patient or the patient's lawful representative.

A physician may testify in court or before a worker's compensation board or the like in any personal injury or related case. (IV)

Issued prior to April 1977.

5.07   Confidentiality: Computers

The utmost effort and care must be taken to protect the confidentiality of all medical records, including computerized medical records.

The guidelines below are offered to assist physicians and computer service organizations in maintaining the confidentiality of information in medical records when that information is stored in computerized data bases:

(1) Confidential medical information should be entered into the computer-based patient record only by authorized personnel. Additions to the record should be time and date stamped, and the person making the additions should be identified in the record.

(2) The patient and physician should be advised about the existence of computerized data bases in which medical information concerning the patient is stored. Such information should be communicated to the physician and patient prior to the physician's release of the medical information to the entity or entities maintaining the computer data bases. All individuals and organizations with some form of access to the computerized data bases, and the level of access permitted, should be specifically identified in advance. Full disclosure of this information to the patient is necessary in obtaining informed consent to treatment. Patient data should be assigned a security level appropriate for the data's degree of sensitivity, which should be used to control who has access to the information.

(3) The physician and patient should be notified of the distribution of all reports reflecting identifiable patient data prior to distribution of the reports by the computer facility. There should be approval by the patient and notification of the physician prior to the release of patient-identifiable clinical and administrative data to individuals or organizations external to the medical care environment. Such information should not be released without the express permission of the patient.

(4) The dissemination of confidential medical data should be limited to only those individuals or agencies with a bona fide use for the data. Only the data necessary for the bona fide use should be released. Patient identifiers should be omitted when appropriate. Release of confidential medical information from the data base should be confined to the specific purpose for which the information is requested and limited to the specific time frame requested. All such organizations or individuals should be advised that authorized release of data to them does not authorize their further release of the data to additional individuals or organizations, or subsequent use of the data for other purposes.

(5) Procedures for adding to or changing data on the computerized data base should indicate individuals authorized to make changes, time periods in which changes take place, and those individuals who will be informed about changes in the data from the medical records.

(6) Procedures for purging the computerized data base of archaic or inaccurate data should be established and the patient and physician should be notified before and after the data has been purged. There should be no mixing of a physician's computerized patient records with those of other computer service bureau clients. In addition, procedures should be developed to protect against inadvertent mixing of individual reports or segments thereof.

(7) The computerized medical data base should be on-line to the computer terminal only when authorized computer programs requiring the medical data are being used. Individuals and organizations external to the clinical facility should not be provided on-line access to a computerized data base containing identifiable data from medical records concerning patients.

Access to the computerized data base should be controlled through security measures such as passwords, encryption (encoding) of information, and scannable badges or other user identification.

(8) Back-up systems and other mechanisms should be in place to prevent data loss and downtime as a result of hardware or software failure.

(9) Security:

(a) Stringent security procedures should be in place to prevent unauthorized access to computer-based patient records. Personnel audit procedures should be developed to establish a record in the event of unauthorized disclosure of medical data. Terminated or former employees in the data processing environment should have no access to data from the medical records concerning patients.

(b) Upon termination of computer services for a physician, those computer files maintained for the physician should be physically turned over to the physician. They may be destroyed (erased) only if it is established that the physician has another copy (in some form). In the event of file erasure, the computer service bureau should verify in writing to the physician that the erasure has taken place. (IV)

Issued prior to April 1977.

Updated June 1994 and June 1998.

5.075 Confidentiality: Disclosure of Records to Data Collection Companies

Data collection from computerized or other patient records for marketing purposes raises serious ethical concerns. In some cases, firms have sought to amass information on physicians' prescribing practices on behalf of pharmaceutical houses for marketing purposes. Often, physicians are offered incentives such as computer hardware and software packages in return for agreeing to such an arrangement. They may be told that data-collecting software does not capture patients' names.

These arrangements may violate principles of informed consent and patient confidentiality. Patients divulge information to their physicians only for purposes of diagnosis and treatment. If other uses are to be made of the information, patients must give their permission after being fully informed about the purpose of such disclosures. If permission is not obtained, physicians violate patient confidentiality by sharing specific and intimate information from patients' records with commercial interests.

Arrangements of this kind may also violate Opinion 8.061, Gifts to Physicians From Industry.

Finally, these arrangements may harm the integrity of the patient-physician relationship. The trust that is fundamental to this relationship is based on the principle that the physicians are the agents first and foremost of their patients. (I, II, IV)

Issued June 1994.

Updated June 1998.

5.08 Confidentiality: Insurance Company Representative

History, diagnosis, prognosis, and the like acquired during the physician-patient relationship may be disclosed to an insurance company representative only if the patient or a lawful representative has consented to the disclosure. A physician's responsibilities to patients are not limited to the actual practice of medicine. They also include the performance of some services ancillary to the practice of medicine. These services might include certification that the patient was under the physician's care and comment on the diagnosis and therapy in the particular case. See also Opinion 2.135. (IV)

Issued prior to April 1977.

5.09   The previous Opinion 5.09, **Confidentiality: Physicians in Industry**, issued July 1983, was deleted in June 2000 and combined with Opinion 5.09.

5.09 Confidentiality: Industry-Employed Physicians and Independent Medical Examiners

Where a physician's services are limited to performing an isolated assessment of an individual's health or disability for an employer, business, or insurer, the information obtained by the physician as a result of such examinations is confidential and should not be communicated to a third party without the individual's prior written consent, unless required by law. If the individual authorized the release of medical information to an employer or a potential employer, the physician should release only that information which is reasonably relevant to the employer's decision regarding that individual's ability to perform the work required by the job.

When a physician renders treatment to an employee, with a work-related illness or injury, the release of medical information to the employer as to the treatment provided may be subject to the provisions of worker's compensation laws. The physician must comply with the requirements of such laws, if applicable. However, the physician may not otherwise discuss the employee's health condition with the employer without the employee's consent or, in the event of the employee's incapacity, the appropriate proxy's consent.

Whenever statistical information about employees' health is released, all employee identities should be deleted. (IV)

Issued December 1999 based on the report "Patient-Physician Relationship in the Context of Work-Related and Independent Medical Examinations," adopted June 1999.

6.00 Opinions on Fees and Charges

6.01 Contingent Physician Fees

If a physician's fee for medical service is contingent on the successful outcome of a claim, such as a malpractice or worker's compensation claim, there is the ever-present danger that the physician may become less of a healer and more of an advocate or partisan in the proceedings. Accordingly, a physician's fee for medical services should be based on the value of the service provided by the physician to the patient and not on the uncertain outcome of a contingency that does not in any way relate to the value of the medical service.

A physician's fee should not be made contingent on the successful outcome of medical treatment. Such arrangements are unethical because they imply that successful outcomes from treatment are guaranteed, thus creating unrealistic expectations of medicine and false promises to consumers. (VI)

Issued prior to April 1977.

Updated June 1994.

6.02 Fee Splitting

Payment by or to a physician solely for the referral of a patient is fee splitting and is unethical.

A physician may not accept payment of any kind, in any form, from any source, such as a pharmaceutical company or pharmacist, an optical company or the manufacturer of medical appliances and devices, for prescribing or referring a patient to said source.

In each case, the payment violates the requirement to deal honestly with patients and colleagues. The patient relies upon the advice of the physician on matters of referral. All referrals and prescriptions must be based on the skill and quality of the physician to whom the patient has been referred or the quality and efficacy of the drug or product prescribed. (II)

Issued prior to April 1977.

Updated June 1994.

6.03 Fee Splitting: Referrals to Health Care Facilities

Clinics, laboratories, hospitals, or other health care facilities that compensate physicians for referral of patients are engaged in fee splitting which is unethical.

Health care facilities should not compensate a physician who refers patients there for the physician's cognitive services in prescribing, monitoring, or revising the patient's course of treatment. Payment for these cognitive services is acceptable when it comes from patients, who are the beneficiaries of the physician's services, or from the patient's designated third-party payer.

Offering or accepting payment for referring patients to research studies (finder's fees) is also unethical. (II)

Issued prior to April 1977.

Updated June 1994 and updated June 1996 based on the report "Finder's Fees: Payment for the Referral of Patients to Clinical Research Studies," adopted December 1994.

6.04   Fee Splitting: Drug or Device Prescription Rebates

A physician may not accept any kind of payment or compensation from a drug company or device manufacturer for prescribing its products. The physician should keep the following considerations in mind:
(1) A physician should only prescribe a drug or device based on reasonable expectations of the effectiveness of the drug or device for the particular patient.
(2) The quantity of the drug prescribed should be no greater than that which is reasonably required for the patient's condition. (II)

Issued March 1980.

6.05   Fees for Medical Services

A physician should not charge or collect an illegal or excessive fee. For example, an illegal fee occurs when a physician accepts an assignment as full payment for services rendered to a Medicare patient and then bills the patient for an additional amount. A fee is excessive when after a review of the facts a person knowledgeable as to current charges made by physicians would be left with a definite and firm conviction that the fee is in excess of a reasonable fee. Factors to be considered as guides in determining the reasonableness of a fee include the following:
(1) the difficulty and/or uniqueness of the services performed and the time, skill, and experience required;
(2) the fee customarily charged in the locality for similar physician services;
(3) the amount of the charges involved;
(4) the quality of performance;
(5) the experience, reputation, and ability of the physician in performing the kind of services involved. (II)

Issued prior to April 1977.

Updated June 1994.

6.06   The previous Opinion 6.06, **Fees: Group Practice**, issued in March 1981, was deleted in June 1994.

6.07   Insurance Form Completion Charges

The attending physician should complete without charge the appropriate "simplified" insurance claim form as a part of service to the patient to enable the patient to receive his or her benefits. A charge for more complex or multiple forms may be made in comformity with local custom. (II)

Issued prior to April 1977.

Updated June 1994.

6.08   Interest Charges and Finance Charges

Although harsh or commercial collection practices are discouraged in the practice of medicine, a physician who has experienced problems with delinquent accounts may properly choose to request that payment be made at the time of treatment or add interest or other reasonable charges to delinquent accounts. The patient must be notified in advance of the interest or other reasonable finance or service charges by such means as the posting of a notice in the physician's waiting room, the distribution of leaflets describing the office billing practices and appropriate notations on the billing statement. The physician must comply with state and federal laws and regulations applicable to the imposition of such charges. Physicians are encouraged to review their accounting/collection policies to ensure that no patient's account is sent to collection without the physician's knowledge. Physicians who choose to add an interest or finance charge to accounts not paid within a reasonable time are encouraged to use compassion and discretion in hardship cases. (II)

Issued prior to April 1977.

Updated June 1994.

6.09   Laboratory Bill

When it is not possible for the laboratory bill to be sent directly to the patient, the referring physician's bill to the patient should indicate the actual charges for laboratory services, including the name of the laboratory, as well as any separate charges for the physician's own professional services. (II)

Issued prior to April 1977.

6.10   Services Provided by Multiple Physicians

Each physician engaged in the care of the patient is entitled to compensation commensurate with the value of the service he or she has personally rendered.

No physician should bill or be paid for a service which is not performed; mere referral does not constitute a professional service for which a professional charge should be made or for which a fee may be ethically paid or received.

When services are provided by more than one physician, each physician should submit his or her own bill to the patient and be compensated separately, if possible. A physician should not charge a markup, commission, or profit on the services rendered by others.

It is ethically permissible in certain circumstances, however, for a surgeon to engage other physicians to assist in the performance of a surgical procedure and to pay a reasonable amount for such assistance, provided the nature of the financial arrangement is made known to the patient. This principle applies whether or not the assisting physician is the referring physician. (II)

Issued prior to April 1977.

Updated June 1994.

6.11 Competition

Competition between and among physicians and other health care practitioners on the basis of competitive factors such as quality of services, skill, experience, miscellaneous conveniences offered to patients, credit terms, fees charged, etc., is not only ethical but is encouraged. Ethical medical practice thrives best under free market conditions when prospective patients have adequate information and opportunity to choose freely between and among competing physicians and alternate systems of medical care. (VII)

Issued July 1983.

6.12 Forgiveness or Waiver of Insurance Co-payments

Under the terms of many health insurance policies or programs, patients are made more conscious of the cost of their medical care through co-payments. By imposing co-payments for office visits and other medical services, insurers hope to discourage unnecessary health care. In some cases, financial hardship may deter patients from seeking necessary care if they would be responsible for a co-payment for the care. Physicians commonly forgive or waive co-payments to facilitate patient access to needed medical care. When a co-payment is a barrier to needed care because of financial hardship, physicians should forgive or waive the co-payment.

A number of clinics have advertised their willingness to provide detailed medical evaluations and accept the insurer's payment but waive the co-payment for all patients. Cases have been reported in which some of these clinics have conducted excessive and unnecessary medical testing while certifying to insurers that the testing is medically necessary. Such fraudulent activity exacerbates the high cost of health care, violates Opinion 2.19, and is unethical.

Physicians should be aware that forgiveness or waiver of co-payments may violate the policies of some insurers, both public and private; other insurers may permit forgiveness or waiver if they are aware of the reasons for the forgiveness or waiver. Routine forgiveness or waiver of co-payments may constitute fraud under state and federal law. Physicians should ensure that their policies on co-payments are consistent with applicable law and with the requirements of their agreements with insurers. (II)

Issued June 1993.

6.13   Professional Courtesy

Professional courtesy refers to the provision of medical care to physician colleagues or their families free of charge or at a reduced rate. While professional courtesy is a long-standing tradition in the medical profession, it is not an ethical requirement. Physicians should use their own judgment in deciding whether to waive or reduce their fees when treating fellow physicians or their families. Physicians should be aware that accepting insurance payments while waiving patient co-payments may violate Opinion 6.12. (II, IV)

Issued June 1994.

7.00 Opinions on Physician Records

7.01 Records of Physicians: Availability of Information to Other Physicians

The interest of the patient is paramount in the practice of medicine, and everything that can reasonably and lawfully be done to serve that interest must be done by all physicians who have served or are serving the patient. A physician who formerly treated a patient should not refuse for any reason to make records of that patient promptly available on request to another physician presently treating the patient. Proper authorization for the use of records must be granted by the patient. Medical reports should not be withheld because of an unpaid bill for medical services. (IV)

Issued prior to April 1977.

7.02 Records of Physicians: Information and Patients

Notes made in treating a patient are primarily for the physician's own use and constitute his or her personal property. However, on request of the patient a physician should provide a copy or a summary of the record to the patient or to another physician, an attorney, or other person designated by the patient.

Most states have enacted statutes that authorize patient access to medical records. These statutes vary in scope and mechanism for permitting patients to review or copy medical records. Access to mental health records, particularly, may be limited by statute or regulation. A physician should become familiar with the applicable laws, rules, or regulations on patient access to medical records.

The record is a confidential document involving the patient-physician relationship and should not be communicated to a third party without the patient's prior written consent, unless required by law or to protect the welfare of the individual or the community. Medical reports should not be withheld because of an unpaid bill for medical services. Physicians may charge a reasonable fee for copying medical records. (IV)

Issued prior to April 1977.

Updated June 1994.

7.025 Records of Physicians: Access by Non-Treating Medical Staff

Physicians who use or receive information from medical records share in the responsibility for preserving patient confidentiality and should play an integral role in the designing of confidentiality safeguards in health care institutions. Physicians have a responsibility to be aware of the appropriate guidelines in their health care institution, as well as the applicable federal and state laws.

Informal case consultations that involve the disclosure of detailed medical information are appropriate in the absence of consent only if the patient cannot be identified from the information.

Only physicians or other health care professionals who are involved in managing the patient, including providing consultative, therapeutic, or diagnostic services, may access the patient's confidential medical information. All others must obtain explicit consent to access the information.

Monitoring user access to electronic or written medical information is an appropriate and desirable means for detecting breaches of confidentiality. Physicians should encourage the development and use of such monitoring systems.

This Opinion focuses on the issue of access to medical records by medical staff not involved in the treatment or diagnosis of patients. It does not address the need to access medical records for clinical research, epidemiological research, quality assurance, or administrative purposes. (IV)

Issued December 1999 based on the report "Records of Physicians: Access by Non-Treating Medical Staff," adopted June 1999.

7.03 Records of Physicians Upon Retirement or Departure from a Group

A patient's records may be necessary to the patient in the future not only for medical care but also for employment, insurance, litigation, or other reasons. When a physician retires or dies, patients should be notified and urged to find a new physician and should be informed that upon authorization, records will be sent to the new physician. Records which may be of value to a patient and which are not forwarded to a new physician should be retained, either by the treating physician, another physician, or such other person lawfully permitted to act as a custodian of the records.

The patients of a physician who leaves a group practice should be notified that the physician is leaving the group. Patients of the physician should also be notified of the physician's new address and offered the opportunity to have their medical records forwarded to the departing physician at his or her new practice. It is unethical to withhold such information upon request of a patient. If the responsibility for notifying patients falls to the departing physician rather than to the group, the group should not interfere with the discharge of these duties by withholding patient lists or other necessary information. (IV)

Issued prior to April 1977.

Updated June 1994 and June 1996.

Sale of a Medical Practice

A physician or the estate of a deceased physician may sell to another physician the elements which comprise his or her practice, such as furniture, fixtures, equipment, office leasehold, and goodwill. In the sale of a medical practice, the purchaser is buying not only furniture and fixtures, but also goodwill, i.e., the opportunity to take over the patients of the seller.

The transfer of records of patients is subject, however, to the following:

(1) All active patients should be notified that the physician (or the estate) is transferring the practice to another physician who will retain custody of their records and that at their written request, within a reasonable time as specified in the notice, the records or copies will be sent to any other physician of their choice. Rather than destroy the records of a deceased physician, it is better that they be transferred to a practicing physician who will retain them subject to requests from patients that they be sent to another physician.

(2) A reasonable charge may be made for the cost of duplicating records. (IV)

Issued July 1983.

Retention of Medical Records

Physicians have an obligation to retain patient records which may reasonably be of value to a patient. The following guidelines are offered to assist physicians in meeting their ethical and legal obligations:

(1) Medical considerations are the primary basis for deciding how long to retain medical records. For example, operative notes and chemotherapy records should always be part of the patient's chart. In deciding whether to keep certain parts of the record, an appropriate criterion is whether a physician would want the information if he or she were seeing the patient for the first time.

(2) If a particular record no longer needs to be kept for medical reasons, the physician should check state laws to see if there is a requirement that records be kept for a minimum length of time. Most states will not have such a provision. If they do, it will be part of the statutory code or state licensing board.

(3) In all cases, medical records should be kept for at least as long as the length of time of the statute of limitations for medical malpractice claims. The statute of limitations may be three or more years, depending on the state law. State medical associations and insurance carriers are the best resources for this information.

(4) Whatever the statute of limitations, a physician should measure time from the last professional contact with the patient.

(5) If a patient is a minor, the statute of limitations for medical malpractice claims may not apply until the patient reaches the age of majority.

(6) Immunization records always must be kept.

(7) The records of any patient covered by Medicare or Medicaid must be kept at least five years.

(8) In order to preserve confidentiality when discarding old records, all documents should be destroyed.

(9) Before discarding old records, patients should be given an opportunity to claim the records or have them sent to another physician, if it is feasible to give them the opportunity. (IV, V)

Issued June 1994.

8.00 Opinions on Practice Matters

8.01 Appointment Charges

A physician may charge a patient for a missed appointment or for one not cancelled 24 hours in advance if the patient is fully advised that the physician will make such a charge. (VI)

Issued prior to April 1977.

Updated June 1994.

8.02   The previous Opinion 8.02, **Clinics**, was deleted in June 1994.

8.02 Ethical Guidelines for Physicians in Management Positions and Other Non-Clinical Roles

Physicians in administrative and other non-clinical roles must put the needs of patients first. At least since the time of Hippocrates, physicians have cultivated the trust of their patients by placing patient welfare before all other concerns. The ethical obligations of physicians are not suspended when a physician assumes a position that does not directly involve patient care. (I, VII)

Issued June 1994 based on the report "Ethical Guidelines for Medical Consultants," adopted December 1992.

Updated June 1998.

8.021 Ethical Obligations of Medical Directors

Assuming a title or position that removes the physician from direct patient-physician relationships does not override professional ethical obligations. The term "medical directors," as used here, refers to physicians who are employed by third-party payers in the health care delivery system (i.e., insurance companies, managed care organizations, self-insured employers) or by entities that perform medical appropriateness determinations on behalf of payers. These types of medical directors have specific functions, such as making coverage determinations, which go beyond mere administrative responsibility. The following stem from this understanding.

Whenever physicians employ professional knowledge and values gained through medical training and practice, and in so doing affect individual or group patient care, they are functioning within the professional sphere of physicians and must uphold ethical obligations, including those articulated by the AMA's *Code of Medical Ethics*.

Medical directors acting within the professional sphere, such as when making decisions regarding medical appropriateness, have an overriding ethical obligation to promote professional medical standards. Adherence to professional medical standards includes:

(1) Placing the interests of patients above other considerations, such as personal interests (*e.g.*, financial incentives) or employer business interests (*e.g.*, profit). This entails applying the plan parameters to each patient equally and engaging in neither discrimination nor favoritism.

(2) Using fair and just criteria when making care-related determinations. This entails contributing professional expertise to help craft plan guidelines that ensure fair and equal consideration of all plan enrollees. In addition, medical directors should review plan policies and guidelines to ensure that decision-making mechanisms are objective, flexible and consistent, and apply only ethically appropriate criteria, such as those identified by the Council in Opinion 2.03, Allocation of Limited Medical Resources.

(3) Working towards achieving access to adequate medical services. This entails encouraging employers to provide services that would be considered part of an adequate level of health care, as articulated in Opinion 2.095, The Provision of Adequate Health Care. (I, III, VII)

Issued December 1999 based on the report "Ethical Obligations of Medical Directors," adopted June 1999.

8.03   Conflicts of Interest: Guidelines

Under no circumstances may physicians place their own financial interests above the welfare of their patients. The primary objective of the medical profession is to render service to humanity; reward or financial gain is a subordinate consideration. For a physician unnecessarily to hospitalize a patient, prescribe a drug, or conduct diagnostic tests for the physician's financial benefit is unethical. If a conflict develops between the physician's financial interest and the physician's responsibilities to the patient, the conflict must be resolved to the patient's benefit. (II)

Issued July 1986.

Updated June 1994.

8.031   Conflicts of Interest: Biomedical Research

Avoidance of real or perceived conflicts of interest in clinical research is imperative if the medical community is to ensure objectivity and maintain individual and institutional integrity. All medical centers should develop specific guidelines for their clinical staff on conflicts of interest. These guidelines should include the following rules: (1) once a clinical investigator becomes involved in a research project for a company or knows that he or she might become involved, she or he, as an individual, cannot ethically buy or sell the company's stock until the involvement ends and the results of the research are published or otherwise disseminated to the public; (2) any remuneration received by the researcher from the company whose product is being studied must be commensurate with the efforts of the researcher on behalf of the company; (3) clinical investigators should disclose any material ties to companies whose products they are investigating including: financial ties, participation in educational activities supported by the companies, participation in other research projects funded by the companies, consulting arrangements, and any other ties. The disclosures should be made in writing to the medical center where the research is conducted, organizations that are funding the research, and journals that publish the results of the research. An explanatory statement that discloses conflicts of interest should accompany all published research. Other types of publications, such as a letters to the editor, should also include an explanatory statement that discloses any potential conflict of interest.

In addition, medical centers should form review committees to examine disclosures by clinical staff about financial associations with commercial corporations. (II, IV)

Issued March 1992 based on the report "Conflicts of Interest in Biomedical Research," adopted December 1989 (JAMA. 1990; 263: 2790-2793).

Updated June 1999 based on the report "Conflicts of Interest: Biomedical Research," adopted December 1998.

8.032 Conflicts of Interest: Health Facility Ownership by a Physician

Physician ownership interests in commercial ventures can provide important benefits in patient care. Physicians are free to enter lawful contractual relationships, including the acquisition of ownership interests in health facilities, products, or equipment. However, when physicians refer patients to facilities in which they have an ownership interest, a potential conflict of interest exists. In general, physicians should not refer patients to a health care facility which is outside their office practice and at which they do not directly provide care or services when they have an investment interest in that facility. The requirement that the physician directly provide the care or services should be interpreted as commonly understood. The physician needs to have personal involvement with the provision of care on site.

There may be situations in which a needed facility would not be built if referring physicians were prohibited from investing in the facility. Physicians may invest in and refer to an outside facility, whether or not they provide direct care or services at the facility, if there is a demonstrated need in the community for the facility and alternative financing is not available. Need might exist when there is no facility of reasonable quality in the community or when use of existing facilities is onerous for patients. Self-referral based on demonstrated need cannot be justified simply if the facility would offer some marginal improvement over the quality of services in the community. The potential benefits of the facility should be substantial. The use of existing facilities may be considered onerous when patients face undue delays in receiving services, delays that compromise the patient's care or affect the curability or reversibility of the patient's condition. The requirement that alternative financing not be available carries a burden of proof. The builder would have to undertake efforts to secure funding from banks, other financial institutions, and venture capitalists before turning to self-referring physicians.

Where there is a true demonstrated need in the community for the facility, the following requirements should also be met: (1) physicians should disclose their investment interest to their patients when making a referral, provide a list of effective alternative facilities if they are available, inform their patients that they have free choice to obtain the medical services elsewhere, and assure their patients that they will not be treated differently if they do not choose the physician-owned facility; (2) individuals not in a position to refer patients to the facility should be given a bona fide opportunity to invest in the facility on the same terms that are offered to referring physicians; (3) the opportunity to invest and the terms of investment should not be related to the past or expected volume of referrals or other business generated by the physician investor or owner; (4) there should be no requirement that a physician investor make referrals to the entity or otherwise generate business as a condition for remaining an investor; (5) the return on the physician's investment should be tied to the physician's equity in the facility rather than to the volume of referrals; (6) the entity should not loan funds or guarantee a loan for physicians in a position to refer to the entity; (7) investment contracts should not include "noncompetition clauses" that prevent physicians from investing in other facilities; (8) the physician's ownership interest should be disclosed to third party payers upon request; (9) an internal utilization review program should be established to ensure that investing physicians do not exploit their patients in any way, as by inappropriate or unnecessary utilization; (10) when a physician's commercial interest conflicts to the detriment of the patient, the physician should make alternative arrangements for the care of the patient. (II, III, IV)

Issued prior to April 1977.

Updated 1989; updated March 1992 based on the report "Conflicts of Interest: Physician Ownership of Medical Facilities," adopted December 1991 (JAMA. 1992; 267: 2366-2369); and updated June 1994.

8.035 Conflicts of Interest in Home Health Care

Physicians who refer patients to home care providers or any other outside facility should avoid possible conflicts of interest by not accepting payment from those providers or facilities for referrals or as compensation for their cognitive services in prescribing, monitoring, or revising a patient's course of treatment. Payment for these cognitive services is acceptable when it comes from patients, who are the beneficiaries of the physician's services, or from the patients' designated third-party payers.

In accordance with Opinion 8.032, physicians may refer patients to home care facilities in which they have an ownership interest if they actively participate on-site in the care provided to patients. Since the appropriate frequency and duration of home visits is a medical decision that should be made on a case-by-case basis, there is no specific minimum number of home visits that may be identified as a conclusive test of the physician's involvement in the patient's home care regimen. Although different patients will have different needs, physicians who directly provide care in the patient's home on at least every fourth visit may presumptively be considered to have made home care a true extension of practice. (II, III, IV)

Issued June 1994 based on the report "Conflicts of Interest: Update on Home Care," adopted December 1993.

Updated 1998.

8.04 Consultation

Physicians should obtain consultation whenever they believe that it would be medically indicated in the care of the patient or when requested by the patient or the patient's representative. When a patient is referred to a consultant, the referring physician should provide a history of the case and such other information as the consultant may need, calling to the attention of the consultant any specific questions about which guidance is sought, and the consultant should advise the referring physician of the results of the consultant's examination and recommendations. (V)

Issued prior to April 1977.

Updated June 1992 and June 1996.

8.041 Second Opinions

Physicians should recommend that a patient obtain a second opinion whenever they believe it would be helpful in the care of the patient. When recommending a second opinion, physicians should explain the reasons for the recommendation and inform their patients that patients are free to choose a second-opinion physician on their own or with the assistance of the first physician. Patients are also free to obtain second opinions on their own initiative, with or without their physician's knowledge.

With the patient's consent, the first physician should provide a history of the case and such other information as the second-opinion physician may need, including the recommendations about management. The second-opinion physician should maintain the confidentiality of the evaluation and should report to the first physician if the consent of the patient has been obtained.

After evaluating the patient, a second-opinion physician should provide the patient with a clear understanding of the opinion, whether or not it agrees with the recommendations of the first physician.

When a patient initiates a second opinion, it is inappropriate for the primary physician to terminate the patient-physician relationship solely because of the patient's decision to obtain a second opinion.

In some cases, patients may ask the second-opinion physician to provide the needed medical care. In general, second-opinion physicians are free to assume responsibility for the care of the patient. It is not unethical to enter into a patient-physician relationship with a patient who has been receiving care from another physician. By accepting second-opinion patients for treatment, physicians affirm the right of patients to have free choice in the selection of their physicians.

There are situations in which physicians may choose not to treat patients for whom they provide second opinions. Physicians may decide not to treat the patient in order to avoid any perceived conflict of interest or loss of objectivity in rendering the requested second opinion. However, the concern about conflicts of interest does not require physicians to decline to treat second-opinion patients. This inherent conflict in the practice of medicine is resolved by the responsible exercise of professional judgment.

Physicians may agree not to treat second-opinion patients as part of their arrangements with insurers or other third party payers. Physicians who enter into such contractual agreements must honor their commitments.

Physicians must decide independently of their colleagues whether to treat second-opinion patients. Physicians may not establish an agreement or understanding among themselves that they will refuse to treat each others' patients when asked to provide a second opinion. Such agreements compromise the ability of patients to receive care from the physicians of their choice and are therefore not only unethical but also unlawful. (IV, V)

Issued June 1992.

Updated June 1996.

8.05 Contractual Relationships

The contractual relationships that physicians assume when they join or affiliate with group practices or agree to provide services to the patients of an insurance plan are varied.

Income arrangements may include hourly wages for physicians working part time, annual salaries for those working full time, and share of group income for physicians who are partners in groups that are somewhat autonomous and contract with plans to provide the required medical care. Arrangements also usually include a range of fringe benefits, such as paid vacations, insurance, and pension plans.

Physicians may work directly for plans or may be employed by the medical group or the hospital that has contracted with the plan to provide services. In the operation of such plans, physicians should not be subjected to lay interference in professional medical matters and their primary responsibility should be to the patients they serve. (VI)

Issued prior to April 1977.

Updated June 1994 and June 1996.

8.051 Conflicts of Interest Under Capitation

The application of capitation to physicians' practices can result in the provision of cost-effective, quality medical care. It is important to note, however, that the potential for conflict exists under such systems. Managed care organizations and the physicians who contract with them should attempt to minimize these conflicts and to ensure that capitation is applied in a manner consistent with the interests of patients.

(1) Physicians have an obligation to evaluate a health plan's capitation payments prior to contracting with that plan to ensure that the quality of patient care is not threatened by inadequate rates of capitation. Capitation payments should be calculated primarily on relevant medical factors, available outcomes data, the costs associated with involved providers, and consensus-oriented standards of necessary care. Furthermore, the predictable costs resulting from existing conditions of enrolled patients should be considered when determining the rate of capitation. Different populations of patients have different medical needs and the costs associated with those needs should be reflected in the per member per month payment. Physicians should seek agreements with plans that provide sufficient financial resources for all necessary care and should refuse to sign agreements that fail in this regard.

(2) Physicians must not assume inordinate levels of financial risk and should therefore consider a number of factors when deciding whether or not to sign a provider agreement. The size of the plan and the time period over which the rate is figured should be considered by physicians evaluating a plan as well as in determinations of the per member per month payment. The capitation rate for large plans can be calculated more accurately than for smaller plans because of the mitigating influence of probability and the behavior of large systems. Similarly, length of time will influence the predictability of patient expenditures and should be considered accordingly. Capitation rates calculated for large plans over an extended period of time are able to be more accurate and are therefore preferable to those calculated for small groups over a short time period.

(3) Stop-loss plans should be in effect to prevent the potential of catastrophic expenses from influencing physician behavior. Physicians should attempt to ensure that such arrangements are finalized prior to signing an agreement to provide services in a health plan.

(4) Physicians must be prepared to discuss with patients any financial arrangements which could impact patient care. Physicians should avoid reimbursement systems that cannot be disclosed to patients without negatively affecting the patient-physician relationship. (II, III, VI)

Issued December 1997 based on the report "The Ethical Implications of Capitation," adopted June 1997.

8.052 Negotiating Discounts for Specialty Care

Patients are entitled to all the benefits outlined in their insurance plan. Therefore, it is unethical for a referring physician to restrict the referral options of patients who have chosen a plan that provides for access to an unlimited or broad selection of specialist physicians. It is also unethical to base the referral of these patients on a discount for the capitated patients in a primary care physician's practice. (II)

Issued December 1997 based on the report "Ethical Issues in Negotiating Discounts for Specialty Care," adopted June 1996.

8.053 Restrictions on Disclosure in Managed Care Contracts

Despite ethical requirements demanding full disclosure of treatment options regardless of limitations imposed by plan coverage, some managed care organizations include clauses in their employment contracts that directly inhibit the ability of physicians to keep their patients fully informed. These types of contract clauses erect inappropriate barriers to necessary communications between physicians and patients, labeled "gag clauses" by some observers. Restrictive clauses of this type impact the ability of physicians to provide information to their patients and to act effectively as a patient advocate. They also threaten to undermine individual and public trust in the profession of medicine.

(1) Managed care organizations have the right to protect proprietary information as long as such protection does not inhibit physicians from disclosing relevant information to patients. Contract clauses that could be applied to prevent physicians from raising or discussing matters relevant to patients' medical care should be removed to safeguard the health of plan subscribers.

(2) The right of patients to be informed of all pertinent medical information must be reaffirmed by the medical profession, and individual physicians must continue to uphold their ethical obligation to disclose such information.

(3) Physicians, individually or through their representative, should review their contracts carefully to ensure that there is no possibility that the health of their patients will be jeopardized in any way by clauses that inhibit their ability to fulfill their ethical obligations. (II, III, VI)

Issued June 1998 based on the report "Restrictions on Disclosure in Managed Care Contracts," adopted June 1996.

8.054 Financial Incentives and the Practice of Medicine

In order to achieve the necessary goals of patient care and to protect the role of physicians as advocates for individual patients, the following statement is offered for the guidance of physicians:

(1) Although physicians have an obligation to consider the needs of broader patient populations within the context of the patient-physician relationship, their first duty must be to the individual patient. This obligation must override considerations of the reimbursement mechanism or specific financial incentives applied to a physician's clinical practice.

(2) Physicians, individually or through their representatives, should evaluate the financial incentives associated with participation in a health plan before contracting with that plan. The purpose of the evaluation is to ensure that the quality of patient care is not compromised by unrealistic expectations for utilization or by placing that physician's payments for care at excessive risk. In the process of making judgments about the ethical propriety of such reimbursement systems, physicians should refer to the following general guidelines:

(a) Monetary incentives may be judged in part on the basis of their size. Large incentives may create conflicts of interest that can in turn compromise clinical objectivity. While an obligation has been established to resolve financial conflicts of interest to the benefit of patients, it is important to recognize that sufficiently large incentives can create an untenable position for physicians;

(b) The proximity of large financial incentives to individual treatment decisions should be limited in order to prevent physicians' personal financial concerns from creating a conflict with their role as individual patient advocates. When the proximity of incentives cannot be mitigated, as in the case of fee-for-service payments, physicians must behave in accordance with prior Council recommendations limiting the potential for abuse. This includes the Council's prohibitions on fee-splitting arrangements, the provision of unnecessary services, unreasonable fees, and self-referral. For incentives that can be distanced from clinical decisions, the following factors should be considered in order to evaluate the correlation between individual act and monetary reward or penalty:

(i) In general, incentives should be applied across broad physician groups. This dilutes the effect any one physician can have on his or her financial situation through clinical recommendations, thus allowing physicians to provide those services they feel are necessary in each case. Simultaneously, however, physicians are encouraged by the incentive to practice efficiently.

(ii) The size of the patient pool considered in calculations of incentive payments will affect the proximity of financial motivations to individual treatment decisions. The laws of probability dictate that in large populations of patients, the overall level of utilization remains relatively stable and predictable. Physicians practicing in plans with large numbers of patients in a risk pool therefore have greater freedom to provide the care they feel is necessary based on the likelihood that the needs of other plan patients will balance out decisions to provide extensive care.

(iii) The time period over which incentives are determined should be long enough to accommodate fluctuations in utilization resulting from the random distribution of patients and illnesses. For example, basing incentive payments on an annual analysis of resource utilization is preferable to basing them on monthly review.

(iv) Financial rewards or penalties that are triggered by specific points of utilization may create enormous incentives as a physician's practice approaches the established level. Incentives should therefore be calculated on a continuum of utilization rather than a bracketed system with tiers of widely varied bonuses or penalties.

    (v) A stop-loss plan should be in place to prevent the costs of treating a single patient from significantly impacting the reward or penalty offered to a physician.

(3) Incentives should be designed to promote efficient practice, but should not be designed to realize cost savings beyond those attainable through efficiency. As a counterbalance to the focus on utilization reduction, incentives should also be based upon measures of quality of care and patient satisfaction.

(4) Patients must be informed of financial incentives that could impact the level or type of care they receive. This responsibility should be assumed by the health plan to ensure that patients are aware of such incentives prior to enrollment. Physicians, individually or through their representatives, must be prepared to discuss with patients any financial arrangements that could impact patient care. Physicians should avoid reimbursement systems that cannot be disclosed to patients without negatively affecting the patient-physician relationship. (II, III)

Issued June 1998 based on the report "Financial Incentives and the Practice of Medicine," adopted December 1997.

8.06   Drugs and Devices: Prescribing

(1) A physician should not be influenced in the prescribing of drugs, devices, or appliances by a direct or indirect financial interest in a pharmaceutical firm or other supplier. Whether the firm is a manufacturer, distributor, wholesaler, or repackager of the products involved is immaterial.

(2) A physician may own or operate a pharmacy but generally may not refer his or her patients to the pharmacy. However, a physician may refer patients to his or her pharmacy if there is a demonstrated need for the pharmacy in the community and alternative financing is unavailable (as defined in Opinion 8.032). Physicians may dispense drugs within their office practices provided there is no resulting exploitation of patients.

(3) A physician should not give patients prescriptions in code or enter into agreements with pharmacies or other suppliers regarding the filling of prescriptions by code.

(4) Patients are entitled to the same freedom of choice in selecting who will fill their prescription needs as they are in the choice of a physician. (See Opinions 9.06 and 8.03.) The prescription is a written direction for a therapeutic or corrective agent. A patient is entitled to a copy of the physician's prescription for drugs, eyeglasses, contact lenses, or other devices as required by the Principles of Medical Ethics and as required by law. The patient has the right to have the prescription filled wherever the patient wishes.

(5) Patients have an ethically and legally recognized right to prompt access to the information contained in their individual medical records. The prescription is an essential part of the patient's medical record. Physicians should not discourage patients from requesting a written prescription or

urge them to fill prescriptions from an establishment which has a direct telephone line or which has entered into a business or other preferential arrangement with the physician with respect to the filling of the physician's prescriptions. (I, II, III, IV, V)

Issued prior to April 1977.

Updated June 1994 based on the report "Conflicts of Interest: Physician Ownership of Medical Facilities," adopted December 1991 (JAMA. 1992; 267: 2366-2369).

8.061 Gifts to Physicians From Industry

Many gifts given to physicians by companies in the pharmaceutical, device, and medical equipment industries serve an important and socially beneficial function. For example, companies have long provided funds for educational seminars and conferences. However, there has been growing concern about certain gifts from industry to physicians. Some gifts that reflect customary practices of industry may not be consistent with the Principles of Medical Ethics. To avoid the acceptance of inappropriate gifts, physicians should observe the following guidelines:

(1) Any gifts accepted by physicians individually should primarily entail a benefit to patients and should not be of substantial value. Accordingly, textbooks, modest meals, and other gifts are appropriate if they serve a genuine educational function. Cash payments should not be accepted.
The use of drug samples for personal or family use is permissible as long as these practices do not interfere with patient access to drug samples. It would not be acceptable for non-retired physicians to request free pharmaceuticals for personal use or use by family members.

(2) Individual gifts of minimal value are permissible as long as the gifts are related to the physician's work (e.g., pens and notepads).

(3) The Council on Ethical and Judicial Affairs defines a legitimate "conference" or "meeting" as any activity, held at an appropriate location, where (a) the gathering is primarily dedicated, in both time and effort, to promoting objective scientific and educational activities and discourse (one or more educational presentation(s) should be the highlight of the gathering), and (b) the main incentive for bringing attendees together is to further their knowledge on the topic(s) being presented. An appropriate disclosure of financial support or conflict of interest should be made.

(4) Subsidies to underwrite the costs of continuing medical education conferences or professional meetings can contribute to the improvement of patient care and therefore are permissible. Since the giving of a subsidy directly to a physician by a company's representative may create a relationship that could influence the use of the company's products, any subsidy should be accepted by the conference's sponsor who in turn can use the money to reduce the conference's registration fee. Payments to defray the costs of a conference should not be accepted directly from the company by the physicians attending the conference.

(5) Subsidies from industry should not be accepted directly or indirectly to pay for the costs of travel, lodging, or other personal expenses of physicians

attending conferences or meetings, nor should subsidies be accepted to compensate for the physicians' time. Subsidies for hospitality should not be accepted outside of modest meals or social events held as a part of a conference or meeting. It is appropriate for faculty at conferences or meetings to accept reasonable honoraria and to accept reimbursement for reasonable travel, lodging, and meal expenses. It is also appropriate for consultants who provide genuine services to receive reasonable compensation and to accept reimbursement for reasonable travel, lodging, and meal expenses. Token consulting or advisory arrangements cannot be used to justify the compensation of physicians for their time or their travel, lodging, and other out-of-pocket expenses.

(6) Scholarship or other special funds to permit medical students, residents, and fellows to attend carefully selected educational conferences may be permissible as long as the selection of students, residents, or fellows who will receive the funds is made by the academic or training institution. Carefully selected educational conferences are generally defined as the major educational, scientific or policy-making meetings of national, regional or specialty medical associations.

(7) No gifts should be accepted if there are strings attached. For example, physicians should not accept gifts if they are given in relation to the physician's prescribing practices. In addition, when companies underwrite medical conferences or lectures other than their own, responsibility for and control over the selection of content, faculty, educational methods, and materials should belong to the organizers of the conferences or lectures. (II)

Issued June 1992 based on the report "Gifts to Physicians from Industry," adopted December 1990 (JAMA. 1991; 265: 501 and *Food and Drug Law Journal*. 1992; 47: 445-458).

Updated June 1996 and June 1998.

8.062 Sale of Non-Health-Related Goods from Physicians' Offices

The sale of non-health-related goods by physicians presents a conflict of interest and threatens to erode the primary obligation of physicians to serve the interests of their patients before their own. Furthermore this activity risks placing undue pressure on the patient and risks demeaning the practice of medicine.

Physicians should not sell non-health-related goods from their offices or other treatment settings, with the exception noted below.

Physicians may sell low-cost non-health-related goods from their offices for the benefit of community organizations, provided that (1) the goods in question are low-cost; (2) the physician takes no share in profit from their sale; (3) such sales are not a regular part of the physician's business; (4) sales are conducted in a dignified manner; and (5) sales are conducted in such a way as to assure that patients are not pressured into making purchases. (I, II)

Issued June 1998 based on the report "Sale of Non-Health-Related Goods from Physicians' Offices," adopted December 1997.

8.063 Sale of Health-Related Products from Physicians' Offices

"Health-related products" are any products that, according to the manufacturer or distributor, benefit health. "Selling" refers to the activity of dispensing items that are provided from the physician's office in exchange for money and also includes the activity of endorsing a product that the patient may order or purchase elsewhere that results in direct remuneration for the physician. This Opinion does not apply to the sale of prescription items which is already addressed in Opinion 8.03, Conflicts of Interest: Guidelines.

Physicians who engage in in-office sales practices should be aware of the related guidelines presented in Opinion 8.062, Sale of Non-Health-Related Goods from Physicians' Offices; Opinion 8.03, Conflicts of Interest: Guidelines; Opinion 8.032, Conflicts of Interest: Health Facility Ownership by a Physician; Opinion 3.01, Nonscientific Practitioners; Opinion 8.20, Invalid Medical Treatment; as well as the Reports from which these Opinions are extracted.

In-office sale of health-related products by physicians presents a financial conflict of interest, risks placing undue pressure on the patient, and threatens to erode patient trust and undermine the primary obligation of physicians to serve the interests of their patients before their own.

(1) Physicians who choose to sell health-related products from their offices should not sell any health-related products whose claims of benefit lack scientific validity. When judging the efficacy of a product, physicians should rely on peer-reviewed literature and other unbiased scientific sources that review evidence in a sound, systematic, and reliable fashion.

(2) Because of the risk of patient exploitation and the potential to demean the profession of medicine, physicians who choose to sell health-related products from their offices must take steps to minimize their financial conflicts of interest. The following guidelines apply:

   (a) In general, physicians should limit sales to products that serve the immediate and pressing needs of their patients. For example, if traveling to the closest pharmacy would in some way jeopardize the welfare of the patient (e.g., forcing a patient with a broken leg to travel to a local pharmacy for crutches), then it may be appropriate to provide the product from the physician's office. These conditions are explained in more detail in the Council's Opinion 8.03, Conflicts of Interest: Guidelines, and are analogous to situations that constitute exceptions to the permissibility of self-referral.

   (b) Physicians may distribute other health-related products to their patients free of charge or at cost, in order to make useful products readily available to their patients. When health-related products are offered free or at cost, it helps to ensure removal of the elements of personal gain and financial conflicts of interest that may interfere, or appear to interfere, with the physician's independent medical judgment.

(3) Physicians must disclose fully the nature of their financial arrangement with a manufacturer or supplier to sell health-related products. Disclosure includes informing patients of financial interests as well as about the availability of the product or other equivalent products elsewhere. Disclosure can be accomplished through face-to-face communication or by posting an easily understandable written notification in a prominent location that is

accessible by all patients in the office. In addition, physicians should, upon request, provide patients with understandable literature that relies on scientific standards in addressing the risks, benefits and limits of knowledge regarding the health-related product.

(4) Physicians should not participate in exclusive distributorships of health-related products which are available only through physicians' offices. Physicians should encourage manufacturers to make products of established benefit more fairly and more widely accessible to patients than exclusive distribution mechanisms allow. (II)

Issued December 1999 based on the report "Sale of Health-Related Products from Physicians' Offices," adopted June 1999.

8.07 Gifts to Physicians: Offers of Indemnity

Physicians should prescribe drugs, devices, and other treatments based solely upon medical considerations and patient needs. A third party's offer to indemnify a physician for lawsuits arising from the physician's prescription or use of the third party's drug, device, or other product, introduces inappropriate factors into medical decision making. Such offers, regardless of their limitations, therefore constitute unacceptable gifts.

This opinion does not address contractual assignments of liability between employers or in research arrangements, nor does it address government indemnification plans. (II)

Issued June 1992 based on the report "Offers of Indemnity by Manufacturers of Drugs, Devices or other Products."

Updated June 1994.

8.08 Informed Consent

The patient's right of self-decision can be effectively exercised only if the patient possesses enough information to enable an intelligent choice. The patient should make his or her own determination on treatment. The physician's obligation is to present the medical facts accurately to the patient or to the individual responsible for the patient's care and to make recommendations for management in accordance with good medical practice. The physician has an ethical obligation to help the patient make choices from among the therapeutic alternatives consistent with good medical practice. Informed consent is a basic social policy for which exceptions are permitted: (1) where the patient is unconscious or otherwise incapable of consenting and harm from failure to treat is imminent; or (2) when risk-disclosure poses such a serious psychological threat of detriment to the patient as to be medically contraindicated. Social policy does not accept the paternalistic view that the physician may remain silent because divulgence might prompt the patient to forego needed therapy. Rational, informed patients should not be expected to act uniformly, even under similar circumstances, in agreeing to or refusing treatment. (I, II, III, IV, V)

Issued March 1981.

Waiver of Informed Consent for Research in Emergency Situations

The current state of emergency medicine and research has resulted in the application of standard treatments that often have not been scientifically evaluated for safety and effectiveness and may render unsatisfactory outcomes. Given the insufficiency of standard treatment alternatives it is appropriate, in certain situations and with special safeguards, to provide experimental treatments without obtaining the informed consent of the subject. However, in order to protect the rights and welfare of the subjects several conditions must be met:

(1) This type of research is limited to emergency, life-threatening situations, and may involve only experimental treatments that are ready for trials involving human subjects.

(2) The subject must lack the capacity to give informed consent for participation in the research.

(3) The window of opportunity for intervention must be so narrow as to make obtaining surrogate consent unfeasible.

(4) Obtaining prospective informed consent for the protocol must not be feasible (*i.e.*, the life threatening emergency situation could not have been anticipated).

(5) The experimental treatment must have a realistic probability of benefit equal to or greater than standard care.

(6) The risks associated with the research should be reasonable in light of the critical nature of the conditions and the risks associated with standard treatment.

(7) Where informed consent is waived, subjects or their representatives must be informed as soon as possible about inclusion in the study and asked to consent to further participation. Subjects, or their representatives, may choose to discontinue participation at any time after being fully informed about the possible consequences. Additionally, if the patient dies while participating in the research protocol, the patient's family or representative must be informed that the patient was involved in an experimental protocol.

(8) Community input should be sought prior to approval of the protocol, and public disclosure should be made of study results. Fair randomization of research subjects should be given thorough consideration. Moreover, an independent data monitoring board should be established to oversee the ongoing trial. (I, V)

Issued December 1997 based on the report "Waiver of Informed Consent for Research in Emergency Situations," adopted June 1997.

Laboratory Services

(1) A physician should not misrepresent or aid in the misrepresentation of laboratory services performed and supervised by a non-physician as the physician's professional services. Such situations could involve a laboratory owned by a physician who directs and manages its financial and business affairs with no professional medical services being provided; laboratory

work being performed by technicians and directly supervised by a medical technologist with no participation by the physician; or the physician's name being used in connection with the laboratory so as to create the appearance that it is owned, operated, and supervised by a physician when this is not so.

(2) If a laboratory is owned, operated, and supervised by a non-physician in accordance with state law and performs tests exclusively for physicians who receive the results and make their own medical interpretations, the following considerations would apply:

The physician's ethical responsibility is to provide patients with high quality services. This includes services that the physician performs personally and those that are delegated to others. A physician should not utilize the services of any laboratory, irrespective of whether it is operated by a physician or non-physician, unless she or he has the utmost confidence in the quality of its services. A physician must always assume personal responsibility for the best interests of his or her patients. Medical judgment based upon inferior laboratory work is likewise inferior. Medical considerations, not cost, must be paramount when the physician chooses a laboratory. The physician who disregards quality as the primary criterion or who chooses a laboratory solely because it provides low cost laboratory services on which the patient is charged a profit, is not acting in the best interests of the patient. However, if reliable, quality laboratory services are available at lower cost, the patient should have the benefit of the savings. As a professional, the physician is entitled to fair compensation for his or her services. A physician should not charge a markup, commission, or profit on the services rendered by others. A markup is an excessive charge that exploits patients if it is nothing more than a tacked on amount for a service already provided and accounted for by the laboratory. A physician may make an acquisition charge or processing charge. The patient should be notified of any such charge in advance. (I, II, III, IV, V)

Issued prior to April 1977.

Updated June 1994.

8.095 Reporting Clinical Test Results: General Guidelines

To alleviate patients' anxieties, physicians should report clinical test results to patients within a reasonable time frame. Since many variables contribute to the urgency of a particular situation, physicians should use their best professional judgment when determining what length of time is reasonable for the particular situation at hand. Anticipated delays should be explained to patients at the time of testing.

Physicians should adopt a consistent reporting policy that accommodates the demands of their practice while at the same time being considerate of patients' anxieties. The reporting policy should be disclosed to patients, for instance when tests are administered, so patients know what to expect. Reporting policies should take into consideration under what circumstances (*e.g.*, all results, only abnormal results, etc.) and by whom (*e.g.*, the laboratory or the physician) test results are appropriately reported to the patient. Any anticipated inconsistencies should be disclosed to patients as soon as they are discovered.

Physicians should provide test results in language understandable to the patient and in the manner deemed most appropriate by the physician. Any information gathered from test results that would be necessary for patients to make intelligent medical decisions and give informed consent on future medical treatments must be disclosed to them.

Physicians should take all appropriate precautions to ensure the confidentiality of test results. Such precautions may include, but are not limited to, not leaving test results on an answering machine, on voice mail or with a third party unless previously given permission to do so by the patient, not delivering test results via electronic mail, and not sending test results through the mail in any form other than a sealed envelope. (II, IV, V)

Issued December 1998 based on the report "Reporting Clinical Test Results: General Guidelines," adopted June 1998.

8.10 Lien Laws

In states where there are lien laws, a physician may file a lien as a means of assuring payment of his or her fee provided the fee is fixed in amount and not contingent on the amount of settlement of the patient's claim against a third party. (I, VI)

Issued prior to April 1977.

8.11 Neglect of Patient

Physicians are free to choose whom they will serve. The physician should, however, respond to the best of his or her ability in cases of emergency where first aid treatment is essential. Once having undertaken a case, the physician should not neglect the patient. (I, VI)

Issued prior to April 1977.

Updated June 1996.

8.115 Termination of the Physician-Patient Relationship

Physicians have an obligation to support continuity of care for their patients. While physicians have the option of withdrawing from a case, they cannot do so without giving notice to the patient, the relatives, or responsible friends sufficiently long in advance of withdrawal to permit another medical attendant to be secured. (I, VI)

Issued June 1996 (formerly included in Opinion 8.11).

8.12　Patient Information

It is a fundamental ethical requirement that a physician should at all times deal honestly and openly with patients. Patients have a right to know their past and present medical status and to be free of any mistaken beliefs concerning their conditions. Situations occasionally occur in which a patient suffers significant medical complications that may have resulted from the physician's mistake or judgment. In these situations, the physician is ethically required to inform the patient of all the facts necessary to ensure understanding of what has occurred. Only through full disclosure is a patient able to make informed decisions regarding future medical care.

Ethical responsibility includes informing patients of changes in their diagnoses resulting from retrospective review of test results or any other information. This obligation holds even though the patient's medical treatment or therapeutic options may not be altered by the new information.

Concern regarding legal liability which might result following truthful disclosure should not affect the physician's honesty with a patient. (I, II, III, IV)

Issued March 1981.

Updated June 1994.

8.13　The previous Opinion 8.13, **Referral of Patients-Disclosure of Limitation,** was changed to Opinion 8.132 in June 1996.

8.13　Managed Care

The expansion of managed care has brought a variety of changes to medicine including new and different reimbursement systems for physicians with complex referral restrictions and benefits packages for patients. Some of these changes have raised concerns that a physician's ability to practice ethical medicine will be adversely affected by the modifications in the system. In response to these concerns, the following points were developed to provide physicians with general guidelines that will assist them in fulfilling their ethical responsibilities to patients given the changes heralded by managed care.

(1) The duty of patient advocacy is a fundamental element of the physician-patient relationship that should not be altered by the system of health care delivery in which physicians practice. Physicians must continue to place the interests of their patients first.

(2) When managed care plans place restrictions on the care that physicians in the plan may provide to their patients, the following principles should be followed:

(a) Any broad allocation guidelines that restrict care and choices—which go beyond the cost/benefit judgments made by physicians as a part of their normal professional responsibilities—should be established at a policy making level so that individual physicians are not asked to engage in bedside rationing.

(b) Regardless of any allocation guidelines or gatekeeper directives, physicians must advocate for any care they believe will materially benefit their patients.

(c) Physicians should be given an active role in contributing their expertise to any allocation process and should advocate for guidelines that are sensitive to differences among patients. Managed care plans should create structures similar to hospital medical staffs that allow physicians to have meaningful input into the plan's development of allocation guidelines. Guidelines for allocating health care should be reviewed on a regular basis and updated to reflect advances in medical knowledge and changes in relative costs.

(d) Adequate appellate mechanisms for both patients and physicians should be in place to address disputes regarding medically necessary care. In some circumstances, physicians have an obligation to initiate appeals on behalf of their patients. Cases may arise in which a health plan has an allocation guideline that is generally fair but in particular circumstances results in unfair denials of care, i.e., denial of care that, in the physician's judgment, would materially benefit the patient. In such cases, the physician's duty as patient advocate requires that the physician challenge the denial and argue for the provision of treatment in the specific case. Cases may also arise when a health plan has an allocation guideline that is generally unfair in its operations. In such cases, the physician's duty as patient advocate requires not only a challenge to any denials of treatment from the guideline but also advocacy at the health plan's policy-making level to seek an elimination or modification of the guideline.

Physicians should assist patients who wish to seek additional, appropriate care outside the plan when the physician believes the care is in the patient's best interests.

(e) Managed care plans must adhere to the requirement of informed consent that patients be given full disclosure of material information. Full disclosure requires that managed care plans inform potential subscribers of limitations or restrictions on the benefits package when they are considering entering the plan.

(f) Physicians also should continue to promote full disclosure to patients enrolled in managed care organizations. The physician's obligation to disclose treatment alternatives to patients is not altered by any limitations in the coverage provided by the patient's managed care plan. Full disclosure includes informing patients of all of their treatment options, even those that may not be covered under the terms of the managed care plan. Patients may then determine whether an appeal is appropriate, or whether they wish to seek care outside the plan for treatment alternatives that are not covered.

(g) Physicians should not participate in any plan that encourages or requires care below minimum professional standards.

(3) When physicians are employed or reimbursed by managed care plans that offer financial incentives to limit care, serious potential conflicts are created between the physicians' personal financial interests and the needs of

their patients. Efforts to contain health care costs should not place patient welfare at risk. Thus, financial incentives are permissible only if they promote the cost-effective delivery of health care and not the withholding of medically necessary care.

(a) Any incentives to limit care must be disclosed fully to patients by plan administrators upon enrollment and at least annually thereafter.

(b) Limits should be placed on the magnitude of fee withholds, bonuses and other financial incentives to limit care. Calculating incentive payments according to the performance of a sizable group of physicians rather than on an individual basis should be encouraged.

(c) Health plans or other groups should develop financial incentives based on quality of care. Such incentives should complement financial incentives based on the quantity of services used.

(4) Patients have an individual responsibility to be aware of the benefits and limitations of their health care coverage. Patients should exercise their autonomy by public participation in the formulation of benefits packages and by prudent selection of health care coverage that best suits their needs. (I, II, III, V)

Issued June 1996 based on the report "Ethical Issues in Managed Care," adopted June 1994 (JAMA. 1995; 273: 330-335).

8.132   Referral of Patients: Disclosure of Limitations

When a physician agrees to provide treatment, he or she thereby enters into a contractual relationship and assumes an ethical obligation to treat the patient to the best of his or her ability. Preferred Provider Organization (PPO) and Health Maintenance Organization (HMO) contracts generally restrict the participating physician's scope of referral to medical specialists, diagnostic laboratories, and hospitals that have contractual arrangements with the PPO and HMO. Some plans also restrict the circumstances under which referrals may be made to contracting medical specialists. If the PPO or HMO does not permit referral to a non-contracting medical specialist or to a diagnostic or treatment facility when the physician believes that the patient's condition requires such services, the physician should so inform the patient so that the patient may decide whether to accept the outside referral at his or her own expense or confine herself or himself to services available within the PPO or HMO. In determining whether treatment or diagnosis requires referral to outside specialty services, the physician should be guided by standards of good medical practice.

Physicians must not deny their patients access to appropriate medical services based upon the promise of personal financial reward, or the avoidance of financial penalties. Because patients must have the necessary information to make informed decisions about their care, physicians have an obligation to assure the disclosure of medically appropriate treatment alternatives, regardless of cost.

Physicians must assure disclosure of any financial inducements that may tend to limit the diagnostic and therapeutic alternatives that are offered to patients or that may tend to limit patients' overall access to care. Physicians may satisfy this obligation by assuring that the managed care plan makes adequate disclosure to patients enrolled in the plan. Physicians should also promote an effective program of peer review to monitor and evaluate the quality of the patient care services within their practice setting. (II, IV)

Issued June 1986.

Updated June 1994 based on the report "Financial Incentives to Limit Care: Ethical Implications for HMOs and IPAs," adopted June 1990.

8.135 Managed Care Cost Containment Involving Prescription Drugs

Managed care organizations establish drug formulary systems so that physicians will supplement medical judgement with cost considerations in drug selection. To ensure optimal patient care, various ethical requirements must be established for formulary application.

(1) Physicians who participate in managed care plans should maintain awareness of plan decisions about drug selection by staying informed about pharmacy and therapeutics (P&T) committee actions and by ongoing personal review of formulary composition. P&T committee members should include independent physician representatives. Mechanisms should be established for ongoing peer review of formulary policy. Physicians who perceive inappropriate influence on formulary development from pharmaceutical industry consolidation should notify the proper regulatory authorities.

(2) Physicians should be particularly vigilant to ensure that formulary decisions adequately reflect the needs of individual patients and that individual needs are not unfairly sacrificed by decisions based on the needs of the average patient. Physicians are ethically required to advocate for additions to the formulary when they think patients would benefit materially and for exceptions to the formulary on a case-by-case basis when justified by the health care needs of particular patients. Mechanisms to appeal formulary exclusions should be established. Other cost-containment mechanisms, including prescription caps and prior authorization, should not unduly burden physicians or patients in accessing optimal drug therapy.

(3) Limits should be placed on the extent to which managed care plans use incentives or pressures to lower prescription drug costs. Financial incentives are permissible when they promote cost-effectiveness, not when they require withholding medically necessary care. Physicians should not be made to feel that they jeopardize their compensation or participation in a managed care plan if they prescribe drugs that are necessary for their patients but that may also be costly. There should be limits on the magnitude of financial incentives, incentives should be calculated according to the practices of a sizeable group of physicians rather than on an individual basis, and incentives based on quality of care rather than cost of care should be used. Prescriptions should not be changed without physicians having a chance to discuss the change with the patient.

(4) Managed care plans should develop and implement educational programs on cost-effective prescribing practices. Such initiatives are preferable to

financial incentives or pressures by health maintenance organizations or hospitals, which can be ethically problematic.

(5) Patients must be informed of the methods used by their managed care plans to limit prescription drug costs. During enrollment, the plan should disclose the existence of formularies, the provisions for cases in which the physician prescribes a drug that is not included in the formulary and the incentives or other mechanisms used to encourage physicians to consider costs when prescribing drugs. In addition, plans should disclose any relationships with pharmaceutical benefit management companies or pharmaceutical companies that could influence the composition of the formulary. If physicians exhaust all avenues to secure a formulary exception for a significantly advantageous drug, they are still obligated to disclose the option of the more beneficial, more costly drug to the patient, so that the patient can decide whether to pay out-of-pocket. (III)

Issued June 1996 based on the report "Managed Care Cost Containment Involving Prescription Drugs," adopted June 1995.

8.137   The previous Opinion 8.137, **Restrictions on Disclosure in Managed Care Contracts**, issued June 1997, was deleted in June 2000 and combined with Opinion 8.053.

8.14   Sexual Misconduct in the Practice of Medicine

Sexual contact that occurs concurrent with the physician-patient relationship constitutes sexual misconduct. Sexual or romantic interactions between physicians and patients detract from the goals of the physician-patient relationship, may exploit the vulnerability of the patient, may obscure the physician's objective judgment concerning the patient's health care, and ultimately may be detrimental to the patient's well-being.

If a physician has reason to believe that non-sexual contact with a patient may be perceived as or may lead to sexual contact, then he or she should avoid the non-sexual contact. At a minimum, a physician's ethical duties include terminating the physician-patient relationship before initiating a dating, romantic, or sexual relationship with a patient.

Sexual or romantic relationships between a physician and a former patient may be unduly influenced by the previous physician-patient relationship. Sexual or romantic relationships with former patients are unethical if the physician uses or exploits trust, knowledge, emotions, or influence derived from the previous professional relationship. (I, II, IV)

Issued December 1989.

Updated March 1992 based on the report "Sexual Misconduct in the Practice of Medicine," adopted December 1990 (JAMA. 1991; 266: 2741-2745).

8.145 Sexual or Romantic Relations Between Physicians and Key Third Parties

Patients are often accompanied by third parties who play an integral role in the patient-physician relationship. The physician interacts and communicates with these individuals and often is in a position to offer them information, advice, and emotional support. The more deeply involved the individual is in the clinical encounter and in medical decision making, the more troubling sexual or romantic contact with the physician would be. This is especially true for individual whose decisions directly impact on the health and welfare of the patient. Key third parties include, but are not limited to, spouses or partners, parents, guardians, and proxies.

Physicians should refrain from sexual or romantic interactions with key third parties when it is based on the use or exploitation of trust, knowledge, influence, or emotions derived from a professional relationship. The following factors should be considered when considering whether a relationship is appropriate: the nature of the patient's medical problem, the length of the professional relationship, the degree of the third party's emotional dependence on the physician, and the importance of the clinical encounter to the third party and the patient. (I, II)

Issued December 1998 based on the report "Sexual or Romantic Relations between Physicians and Key Third Parties," adopted June 1998.

8.15 Substance Abuse

It is unethical for a physician to practice medicine while under the influence of a controlled substance, alcohol, or other chemical agents which impair the ability to practice medicine. (I)

Issued December 1986.

8.16 Substitution of Surgeon Without Patient's Knowledge or Consent

A surgeon who allows a substitute to operate on his or her patient without the patient's knowledge and consent is deceitful. The patient is entitled to choose his or her own physician and should be permitted to acquiesce to or refuse the substitution.

The surgeon's obligation to the patient requires the surgeon to perform the surgical operation: (1) within the scope of authority granted by the consent to the operation; (2) in accordance with the terms of the contractual relationship; (3) with complete disclosure of facts relevant to the need and the performance of the operation; and (4) utilizing best skill.

It should be noted that it is the operating surgeon to whom the patient grants consent to perform the operation. The patient is entitled to the services of the particular surgeon with whom he or she contracts. The operating surgeon, in accepting the patient, is obligated to utilize his or her personal talents in the performance of the operation to the extent required by the agreement creating the physician-patient relationship. The surgeon cannot properly delegate to another the duties which he or she is required to perform personally.

Under the normal and customary arrangement with patients, and with reference to the usual form of consent to operation, the operating surgeon is obligated to perform the operation but may be assisted by residents or other surgeons. With the consent of the patient, it is not unethical for the operating surgeon to delegate the performance of certain aspects of the operation to the assistant provided this is done under the surgeon's participatory supervision, i.e., the surgeon must scrub. If a resident or other physician is to perform the operation under non-participatory supervision, it is necessary to make a full disclosure of this fact to the patient, and this should be evidenced by an appropriate statement contained in the consent. Under these circumstances, it is the resident or other physician who becomes the operating surgeon. (I, II, IV, V)

Issued prior to April 1977.

Updated June 1994.

8.17 Use of Restraints

All individuals have a fundamental right to be free from unreasonable bodily restraint. Physical and chemical restraints should therefore be used only in the best interest of the patient and in accordance with the following guidelines:

(1) The use of restraints, except in emergencies, may be implemented only upon the explicit order of a physician, in conformance with reasonable professional judgment.

(2) Judgment should be exercised in issuing pro re nata (PRN) orders for the use of physical or chemical restraints, and the implementation of such orders should be frequently reviewed and documented by the physician.

(3) The use of restraints should not be punitive, nor should they be used for convenience or as an alternative to reasonable staffing.

(4) Restraints should be used only in accordance with appropriate clinical indications.

(5) As with all therapeutic interventions, informed consent by the patient or surrogate decision maker is a key element in the application of physical and chemical restraints, and should be incorporated into institutional policy.

(6) In certain limited situations, it may be appropriate to restrain a patient involuntarily. For example, restraints may be needed for the safety of the patient or others in the area. When restraints are used involuntarily, the restraints should be removed when they are no longer needed. (I, IV)

Issued March 1992 based on the report "Guidelines for the Use of Restraints in Long Term Care Facilities," adopted June 1989.

8.18 Informing Families of a Patient's Death

Disclosing the death of a patient to the patient's family is a duty which goes to the very heart of the physician-patient relationship and should not be readily delegated to others by the attending physician. The emotional needs of the family and the integrity of the physician-patient relationship must at all times be given foremost consideration.

Physicians in residency training may be asked to participate in the communication of information about a patient's death, if that request is commensurate with the physician's prior training or experience and previous close personal relationship with the family.

It would not be appropriate for the attending physician or resident to request that a medical student notify family members of a patient's death. Medical students should be trained in issues of death and dying, and should be encouraged to accompany attending physicians when news of a patient's death is conveyed to the family members. (I, IV)

Issued March 1992 based on the report "Informing Families of a Patient's Death: Guidelines for the Involvement of Medical Students," adopted December 1989.

Updated June 1994.

8.19 Self-Treatment or Treatment of Immediate Family Members

Physicians generally should not treat themselves or members of their immediate families. Professional objectivity may be compromised when an immediate family member or the physician is the patient; the physician's personal feelings may unduly influence his or her professional medical judgment, thereby interfering with the care being delivered. Physicians may fail to probe sensitive areas when taking the medical history or may fail to perform intimate parts of the physical examination. Similarly, patients may feel uncomfortable disclosing sensitive information or undergoing an intimate examination when the physician is an immediate family member. This discomfort is particularly the case when the patient is a minor child, and sensitive or intimate care should especially be avoided for such patients. When treating themselves or immediate family members, physicians may be inclined to treat problems that are beyond their expertise or training. If tensions develop in a physician's professional relationship with a family member, perhaps as a result of a negative medical outcome, such difficulties may be carried over into the family member's personal relationship with the physician.

Concerns regarding patient autonomy and informed consent are also relevant when physicians attempt to treat members of their immediate family. Family members may be reluctant to state their preference for another physician or decline a recommendation for fear of offending the physician. In particular, minor children will generally not feel free to refuse care from their parents. Likewise, physicians may feel obligated to provide care to immediate family members even if they feel uncomfortable providing care.

It would not always be inappropriate to undertake self-treatment or treatment of immediate family members. In emergency settings or isolated settings where there is no other qualified physician available, physicians should not hesitate to treat themselves or family members until another physician becomes available. In addition, while physicians should not serve as a primary or regular care provider for immediate family members, there are situations in which routine care is acceptable for short-term, minor problems.

Except in emergencies, it is not appropriate for physicians to write prescriptions for controlled substances for themselves or immediate family members. (I, II, IV)

Issued June 1993.

8.20   Invalid Medical Treatment

The following general guidelines are offered to serve physicians when they are called upon to decide among treatments:

(1) Treatments which have no medical indication and offer no possible benefit to the patient should not be used (Opinion 2.035).

(2) Treatments which have been determined scientifically to be invalid should not be used (Opinion 3.01).

(3) Among the treatments that are scientifically valid, medically indicated, and offer a reasonable chance of benefit for patients, some are regulated or prohibited by law; physicians should comply with these laws. If physicians disagree with such laws, they should seek to change them.

(4) Among the various treatments that are scientifically valid, medically indicated, legal, and offer a reasonable chance of benefit for patients, the decision of which treatment to use should be made between the physician and patient. (I, III, IV)

Issued June 1998 based on the report "Invalid Medical Treatment," adopted December 1997.

8.21   Use of Chaperones During Physical Exams

From the standpoint of ethics and prudence, the protocol of having chaperones available on a consistent basis for patient examinations is recommended. Physicians aim to respect the patient's dignity and to make a positive effort to secure a comfortable and considerate atmosphere for the patient—such actions include the provision of appropriate gowns, private facilities for undressing, sensitive use of draping, and clear explanations on various components of the physical examination. A policy that patients are free to make a request for a chaperone should be established in each health care setting. This policy should be communicated to patients, either by means of a well displayed notice or preferably through a conversation initiated by the intake nurse or the physician. The request by a patient to have a chaperone should be honored.

An authorized health professional should serve as a chaperone whenever possible. In their practices, physicians should establish clear expectations about respecting patient privacy and confidentiality to which chaperones must adhere.

If a chaperone is to be provided, a separate opportunity for private conversation between the patient and the physician should be allowed. The physician should keep inquiries and history-taking, especially those of a sensitive nature, to a minimum during the course of the chaperoned examination. (I, IV)

Issued December 1998 based on the report "Use of Chaperones During Physical Exams," adopted June 1998.

Opinions on Professional Rights and Responsibilities

9.01 Accreditation

Physicians who engage in activities that involve the accreditation, approval, or certification of institutions, facilities, and programs that provide patient care or medical education or certify the attainment of specialized professional competence have the ethical responsibility to apply standards that are relevant, fair, reasonable, and nondiscriminatory. The accreditation of institutions and facilities that provide patient care should be based upon standards that focus upon the quality of patient care achieved. Standards used in the accreditation of patient care and medical education, or the certification of specialized professional attainment should not be adopted or used as a means of economic regulation. (II, IV, VII)

Issued December 1982.

9.011 Continuing Medical Education

Physicians should strive to further their medical education throughout their careers, for only by participating in continuing medical education (CME) can they continue to serve patients to the best of their abilities and live up to professional standards of excellence. Fulfillment of mandatory state CME requirements does not necessarily fulfill the physician's ethical obligation to maintain his or her medical expertise.

Attendees. Guidelines for physicians attending a CME conference or activity are as follows:
(1) The physician choosing among CME activities should assess their educational value and select only those activities which are of high quality and appropriate for the physician's educational needs. When selecting formal CME activities, the physician should, at a minimum, choose only those activities that (a) are offered by sponsors accredited by the Accreditation Council for Continuing Medical Education (ACCME), the American Academy of Family Physicians (AAFP), or a state medical society; (b) contain information on subjects relevant to the physician's needs; (c) are responsibly conducted by qualified faculty; (d) conform to Opinion 8.061, Gifts to Physicians from Industry.

(2) The educational value of the CME conference or activity must be the primary consideration in the physician's decision to attend or participate. Though amenities unrelated to the educational purpose of the activity may play a role in the physician's decision to participate, this role should be secondary to the educational content of the conference.

(3) Physicians should claim credit commensurate with only the actual time spent attending a CME activity or in studying a CME enduring material.

(4) Attending promotional activities put on by industry or their designees is not unethical as long as the conference conforms to Opinion 8.061, Gifts to Physicians from Industry, and is clearly identified as promotional to all participants.

Faculty. Guidelines for physicians serving as presenters, moderators, or other faculty at a CME conference are as follows:

(1) Physicians serving as presenters, moderators, or other faculty at a CME conference should ensure that (a) research findings and therapeutic recommendations are based on scientifically accurate, up-to-date information and are presented in a balanced, objective manner; (b) the content of their presentation is not modified or influenced by representatives of industry or other financial contributors, and they do not employ materials whose content is shaped by industry. Faculty may, however, use scientific data generated from industry-sponsored research, and they may also accept technical assistance from industry in preparing slides or other presentation materials, as long as this assistance is of only nominal monetary value and the company has no input in the actual content of the material.

(2) When invited to present at non-CME activities that are primarily promotional, faculty should avoid participation unless the activity is clearly identified as promotional in its program announcements and other advertising.

(3) All conflicts of interest or biases, such as a financial connection to a particular commercial firm or product, should be disclosed by faculty members to the activity's sponsor and to the audience. Faculty may accept reasonable honoraria and reimbursement for expenses in accordance with Opinion 8.061, Gifts to Physicians from Industry.

Sponsors. Guidelines for physicians involved in the sponsorship of CME activities are as follows:

(1) Physicians involved in the sponsorship of CME activities should ensure that (a) the program is balanced, with faculty members presenting a broad range of scientifically supportable viewpoints related to the topic at hand; (b) representatives of industry or other financial contributors do not exert control over the choice of moderators, presenters, or other faculty, or modify the content of faculty presentations. Funding from industry or others may be accepted in accordance with Opinion 8.061, Gifts to Physicians from Industry.

(2) Sponsors should not promote CME activities in a way that encourages attendees to violate the guidelines of the Council on Ethical and Judicial Affairs, including Opinion 8.061, Gifts to Physicians from Industry, or the principles established for the American Medical Association's Physician

Recognition Award. CME activities should be developed and promoted consistent with guideline (2) for Attendees.

(3) Any non-CME activity that is primarily promotional must be identified as such to faculty and participants, both in its advertising and at the conference itself.

(4) The entity presenting the program should not profit unfairly or charge a fee which is excessive for the content and length of the program.

(5) The program, content, duration, and ancillary activities should be consistent with the ideals of the AMA CME program. (I, V)

Issued December 1993.

Updated June 1996.

9.012 Physicians' Political Communications with Patients and Their Families

Physicians enjoy the rights and privileges of free political speech shared by all Americans. It is laudable for physicians to run for political office, to lobby for political positions, parties or candidates, and in every other way to exercise the full scope of their political rights as citizens. These rights may be exercised individually or through involvement with organizations such as professional societies and political action committees.

In addition, physicians have a responsibility to work for the reform of, and to press for the proper administration of, laws that are related to health care. Physicians should keep themselves well-informed as to current political questions regarding needed and proposed changes to laws concerning such issues as access to health care, quality of health care services, scope of medical research, and promotion of public health.

It is natural that in fulfilling these political responsibilities, physicians will express their views to patients or their families. However, communications by telephone or other modalities with patients and their families about political matters must be conducted with the utmost sensitivity to patients' vulnerability and desire for privacy. Conversations about political matters are not appropriate at times when patients or families are emotionally pressured by significant medical circumstances. Physicians are best able to judge both the intrusiveness of the discussion and the patient's level of comfort. In general, when conversation with the patient or family concerning social, civic, or recreational matters is acceptable, discussion of items of political import may be appropriate.

Under no circumstances should physicians allow their differences with patients or their families about political matters to interfere with the delivery of high quality professional care. (I, VII)

Issued June 1999 based on the report "Physicians' Political Communications with Patients and Their Families," adopted December 1998.

9.02   The previous Opinion 9.02, **Agreements Restricting the Practice of Medicine**, was deleted in June 1998 and replaced with the current Opinion.

9.02   Restrictive Covenants and the Practice of Medicine

Covenants-not-to-compete restrict competition, disrupt continuity of care, and potentially deprive the public of medical services. The Council on Ethical and Judicial Affairs discourages any agreement which restricts the right of a physician to practice medicine for a specified period of time or in a specified area upon termination of an employment, partnership or corporate agreement. Restrictive covenants are unethical if they are excessive in geographic scope or duration in the circumstances presented, or if they fail to make reasonable accommodation of patients' choice of physician. (VI, VII)

Issued prior to April 1977.

Updated June 1994 and June 1998.

9.021   Covenants-Not-to-Compete for Physicians-in-Training

It is unethical for a teaching institution to seek a non-competition guarantee in return for fulfilling its educational obligations. Physicians-in-training (residents in programs approved by the Accreditation Council for Graduate Medical Education (ACGME), fellows in ACGME-approved fellowship programs, and fellows in programs approved by one of the American Board of Medical Specialties specialty boards) should not be asked to sign covenants-not-to-compete as a condition of their entry into any residency or fellowship program. (III, IV, VI)

Issued December 1997 based on the report "Covenants-Not-to-Compete for Physicians-in-Training," adopted June 1997.

9.025   Collective Action and Patient Advocacy

Collective action should not be conducted in a manner that jeopardizes the health and interests of patients. Formal unionization of physicians and physicians-in-training may tie physicians' interests to the interests of workers who may not share physicians' primary and overriding commitment to patients and the public health. Physicians should not form workplace alliances with those who do not share these ethical priorities.

Strikes reduce access to care, eliminate or delay necessary care, and interfere with continuity of care. Each of these consequences is contrary to the physician's ethic. Physicians should refrain from the use of the strike as a bargaining tactic.

There are some measures of collective action that may not impinge on essential patient care. Collective activities aimed at ultimately improving patient care may be warranted in some circumstances, even if they create inconvenience for the management.

Physicians and physicians-in-training should take full advantage of the tools of collective action through which to press for needed reforms. Informational campaigns, non-disruptive public demonstrations, lobbying and publicity campaigns, and collective negotiation are among the options available which do not limit services to patients.

Physicians' collective activities should be in conformance with the law. (I, III)

Issued December 1998 based on the report "Collective Action and Patient Advocacy," adopted June 1998.

9.03 Civil Rights and Professional Responsibility

Opportunities in medical society activities or membership, medical education and training, employment, and all other aspects of professional endeavors should not be denied to any duly licensed physician because of race, color, religion, creed, ethnic affiliation, national origin, sex, sexual orientation, age, or handicap. (IV)

Issued prior to April 1977.

Updated June 1994.

9.031 Reporting Impaired, Incompetent, or Unethical Colleagues

Physicians have an ethical obligation to report impaired, incompetent, and unethical colleagues in accordance with the legal requirements in each state and assisted by the following guidelines:

Impairment. Impairment should be reported to the hospital's in-house impairment program, if available. Otherwise, either the chief of an appropriate clinical service or the chief of the hospital staff should be alerted. Reports may also be made directly to an external impaired physician program. Practicing physicians who do not have hospital privileges should be reported directly to an impaired physician program, such as those run by medical societies, when appropriate. If none of these steps would facilitate the entrance of the impaired physician into an impairment program, then the impaired physician should be reported directly to the state licensing board.

Incompetence. Initial reports of incompetence should be made to the appropriate clinical authority who would be empowered to assess the potential impact on patient welfare and to facilitate remedial action. The hospital peer review body should be notified where appropriate. Incompetence which poses an immediate threat to the health of patients should be reported directly to the state licensing board. Incompetence by physicians without a hospital affiliation should be reported to the local or state medical society and/or the state licensing or disciplinary board.

Unethical conduct. With the exception of incompetence or impairment, unethical behavior should be reported in accordance with the following guidelines:

Unethical conduct that threatens patient care or welfare should be reported to the appropriate authority for a particular clinical service. Unethical behavior which violates state licensing provisions should be reported to the state licensing board or impaired physician programs, when appropriate. Unethical conduct which violates criminal statutes must be reported to the appropriate law enforcement authorities. All other unethical conduct should be reported to the local or state medical society.

Where the inappropriate behavior of a physician continues despite the initial report(s), the reporting physician should report to a higher or additional authority. The person or body receiving the initial report should notify the reporting physician when appropriate action has been taken. Physicians who receive reports of inappropriate behavior have an ethical duty to critically and objectively evaluate the reported information and to assure that identified deficiencies are either remedied or further reported to a higher or additional authority. Anonymous reports should receive appropriate review and confidential investigation. Physicians who are under scrutiny or charge should be protected by the rules of confidentiality until such charges are proven or until the physician is exonerated. (II)

Issued March 1992 based on the report "Reporting Impaired, Incompetent, or Unethical Colleagues," adopted December 1991.

Updated June 1994 and June 1996.

9.032 Reporting Adverse Drug or Device Events

A physician who suspects the occurrence of an adverse reaction to a drug or medical device has an obligation to communicate that information to the broader medical community, (e.g., through submitting a report or letter to a medical journal or informing the manufacturer of the suspect drug or device). In the case of a serious adverse event, the event should be reported to the Food and Drug Administration (FDA). Spontaneous reports of adverse events are irreplaceable as a source of valuable information about drugs and medical devices, particularly their rare or delayed effects, as well as their safety in vulnerable patient populations. Although premarketing and mandated postmarketing studies provide basic safeguards for the public health, they suffer from inherent deficiencies that limit their ability to detect rare or unexpected consequences of drug or medical device use. Physicians who prescribe and monitor the use of drugs and medical devices constitute the group best able to observe and communicate information about resulting adverse events.

Serious adverse events, such as those resulting in death, hospitalization, or medical or surgical intervention, are the most important to report and are the only adverse events for which the FDA desires a report. Certainty, or even reasonable likelihood, of a causal relationship between the drug or medical device and the serious adverse event will rarely exist and is not required before reporting the event to the FDA. Suspicion of such a relationship is sufficient to give rise to an obligation to participate in the reporting system. (I, V, VII)

Issued June 1993 based on the report "Reporting Adverse Drug and Medical Device Events," adopted June 1993.

Updated June 1994.

9.035 Gender Discrimination in the Medical Profession

Physician leaders in medical schools and other medical institutions should take immediate steps to increase the number of women in leadership positions as such positions become open. There is already a large enough pool of female physicians to provide strong candidates for such positions. Also, adjustments should be made to ensure that all physicians are equitably compensated for their work. Women and men in the same specialty with the same experience and doing the same work should be paid the same compensation.

Physicians in the workplace should actively develop the following: (1) retraining or other programs which facilitate the re-entry of physicians who take time away from their careers to have a family; (2) on-site child care services for dependent children; and (3) policies providing job security for physicians who are temporarily not in practice due to pregnancy or family obligations.

Physicians in the academic medical setting should strive to promote the following: (1) extension of tenure decisions through "stop the clock" programs, relaxation of the seven year rule, or part-time appointments that would give faculty members longer to achieve standards for promotion and tenure; (2) more reasonable guidelines regarding the appropriate quantity and timing of published material needed for promotion or tenure that would emphasize quality over quantity and that would encourage the pursuit of careers based on individual talent rather than tenure standards that undervalue teaching ability and overvalue research; and (3) fair distribution of teaching, clinical, research, administrative responsibilities, and access to tenure tracks between men and women. Also, physicians in academic institutions should consider formally structuring the mentoring process, possibly matching students or faculty with advisors through a fair and visible system.

Where such policies do not exist or have not been followed, all medical workplaces and institutions should create strict policies to deal with sexual harassment. Grievance committees should have broad representation of both sexes and other groups. Such committees should have the power to enforce harassment policies and be accessible to those persons they are meant to serve.

Grantors of research funds and editors of scientific or medical journals should consider blind peer review of grant proposals and articles for publication to help prevent bias. However, grantors and editors will be able to consider the author's identity and give it appropriate weight. (II, VII)

Issued June 1994 based on the report "Gender Discrimination in the Medical Profession," adopted June 1993.

9.04 Discipline and Medicine

Incompetence, corruption, or dishonest or unethical conduct on the part of members of the medical profession is reprehensible. In addition to posing a real or potential threat to patients, such conduct undermines the public's confidence in the profession. A physician should expose, without fear or loss of favor, incompetent or corrupt, dishonest or unethical conduct on the part of members of the profession. Questions of such conduct should be reported and reviewed in accordance with Opinion 9.031, Reporting Impaired, Incompetent, or Unethical Colleagues.

Violation of governmental laws may subject the physician to civil or criminal liability. Expulsion from membership is the maximum penalty that may be imposed by a medical society upon a physician who violates the ethical standards involving a breach of moral duty or principle. However, medical societies have a civic and professional obligation to report to the appropriate governmental body or state board of medical examiners credible evidence that may come to their attention involving the alleged criminal conduct of any physician relating to the practice of medicine.

Although a physician charged with allegedly illegal conduct may be acquitted or exonerated in civil or criminal proceedings, this does not discharge a medical society from its obligation to initiate a disciplinary proceeding against a member with reference to the same conduct where there is credible evidence tending to establish unethical conduct.

The Council cannot pass judgment in advance on a situation that may later come before it on appeal. The Council cannot be an attorney for a society or a member thereof and later judge in the same factual situation. The local medical society has the initial obligation of determining all the facts and whether or not disciplinary action is indicated. Questions asking for a review of a proposed course of action or an evaluation of an existing factual situation should be presented to the appropriate official of the physician's local society. (II, III, VII)

Issued prior to April 1977.

Updated June 1994.

9.05   Due Process

The basic principles of a fair and objective hearing should always be accorded to the physician or medical student whose professional conduct is being reviewed. The fundamental aspects of a fair hearing are a listing of specific charges, adequate notice of the right of a hearing, the opportunity to be present and to rebut the evidence, and the opportunity to present a defense. These principles apply when the hearing body is a medical society tribunal, medical staff committee, or other similar body composed of peers. The composition of committees sitting in judgment of medical students, residents, or fellows should include a significant number of persons at a similar level of training.

These principles of fair play apply in all disciplinary hearings and in any other type of hearing in which the reputation, professional status, or livelihood of the physician or medical student may be negatively impacted.

All physicians and medical students are urged to observe diligently these fundamental safeguards of due process whenever they are called upon to serve on a committee which will pass judgment on a peer. All medical societies and institutions are urged to review their constitutions and bylaws and/or policies to make sure that these instruments provide for such procedural safeguards. (II, III, VII)

Issued prior to April 1977.

Updated June 1994.

9.055   Disputes Between Medical Supervisors and Trainees

Clear policies for handling complaints from medical students, resident physicians, and other staff should be established. These policies should include adequate provisions for protecting the confidentiality of complainants whenever possible. Confidentiality of complainants should be protected when doing so does not hinder the subject's ability to respond to the complaint. Access to employment and evaluation files should be carefully monitored to remove the possibility of tampering. Resident physicians should be permitted access to their employment files and also the right to copy the contents thereof, within the provisions of applicable federal and state laws.

Medical students, resident physicians, and other staff should refuse to participate in patient care ordered by their supervisors in those rare cases in which they believe the orders reflect serious errors in clinical or ethical judgment, or physician impairment, that could result in a threat of imminent harm to the patient or to others. In these rare cases, the complainant may withdraw from the care ordered by the supervisor, provided withdrawal does not itself threaten the patient's immediate welfare. The complainant should communicate his or her concerns to the physician issuing the orders and, if necessary, to the appropriate persons for mediating such disputes. Mechanisms for resolving these disputes, which require immediate resolution, should be in place. Third-party mediators of such disputes may include the chief of staff or the involved service, the chief resident, a designated member of the institutional grievance committee, or, in large institutions, an institutional ombudsperson largely outside of the established hospital staff hierarchy.

Retaliatory or punitive actions against those who raise complaints are unethical and are a legitimate cause for filing a grievance with the appropriate institutional committee. (II, III, VII)

Issued June 1994 based on the report "Disputes Between Medical Supervisors and Trainees," adopted December 1993 (JAMA. 1994; 272: 1861-1865).

9.06   Free Choice

Free choice of physicians is the right of every individual. One may select and change at will one's physicians, or one may choose a medical care plan such as that provided by a closed panel or group practice or health maintenance or service organization. The individual's freedom to select a preferred system of health care and free competition among physicians and alternative systems of care are prerequisites of ethical practice and optimal patient care.

In choosing to subscribe to a health maintenance or service organization or in choosing or accepting treatment in a particular hospital, the patient is thereby accepting limitations upon free choice of medical services.

The need of an individual for emergency treatment in cases of accident or sudden illness may, as a practical matter, preclude free choice of a physician, particularly where there is loss of consciousness.

Although the concept of free choice assures that an individual can generally choose a physician, likewise a physician may decline to accept that individual as a patient. In selecting the physician of choice, the patient may sometimes be obliged to pay for medical services which might otherwise be paid by a third party. (IV)

Issued prior to April 1977.

9.065   Caring for the Poor

Each physician has an obligation to share in providing care to the indigent. The measure of what constitutes an appropriate contribution may vary with circumstances such as community characteristics, geographic location, the nature of the physician's practice and specialty, and other conditions. All physicians should work to ensure that the needs of the poor in their communities are met. Caring for the poor should be a regular part of the physician's practice schedule.

In the poorest communities, it may not be possible to meet the needs of the indigent for physicians' services by relying solely on local physicians. The local physicians should be able to turn for assistance to their colleagues in prosperous communities, particularly those in close proximity.

Physicians are meeting their obligation, and are encouraged to continue to do so, in a number of ways such as seeing indigent patients in their offices at no cost or at reduced cost, serving at freestanding or hospital clinics that treat the poor, and participating in government programs that provide health care to the poor. Physicians can also volunteer their services at weekend clinics for the poor and at shelters for battered women or the homeless.

In addition to meeting their obligation to care for the indigent, physicians can devote their energy, knowledge, and prestige to designing and lobbying at all levels for better programs to provide care for the poor. (I, VII)

Issued June 1994 based on the report "Caring for the Poor," adopted December 1992 (JAMA. 1993; 269: 2533-2537).

9.07   Medical Testimony

As a citizen and as a professional with special training and experience, the physician has an ethical obligation to assist in the administration of justice. If a patient who has a legal claim requests a physician's assistance, the physician should furnish medical evidence, with the patient's consent, in order to secure the patient's legal rights.

Medical experts should have recent and substantive experience in the area in which they testify and should limit testimony to their sphere of medical expertise. Medical witnesses should be adequately prepared and should testify honestly and truthfully to the best of their medical knowledge.

The medical witness must not become an advocate or a partisan in the legal proceeding. The medical witness should be adequately prepared and should testify honestly and truthfully. The attorney for the party who calls the physician as a witness should be informed of all favorable and unfavorable information developed by the physician's evaluation of the case. It is unethical for a physician to accept compensation that is contingent upon the outcome of litigation.

(II, IV, V, VII)

Issued June 1986.

Updated June 1996 based on the report "Ethical Guidelines for Medical Experts," adopted December 1995.

9.08 New Medical Procedures

In the ethical tradition expressed by Hippocrates and continuously affirmed thereafter, the role of the physician has been that of a healer who serves patients, a teacher who imparts knowledge of skills and techniques to colleagues, and a student who constantly seeks to keep abreast of new medical knowledge.

Physicians have an obligation to share their knowledge and skills and to report the results of clinical and laboratory research. Both positive and negative studies should be included even though they may not support the author's hypothesis. This tradition enhances patient care, leads to the early evaluation of new technologies, and permits the rapid dissemination of improved techniques.

The intentional withholding of new medical knowledge, skills, and techniques from colleagues for reasons of personal gain is detrimental to the medical profession and to society and is to be condemned.

Prompt presentation before scientific organizations and timely publication of clinical and laboratory research in scientific journals are essential elements in the foundation of good medical care. (I, II, V, VII)

Issued December 1984.

Updated June 1994.

9.09 Patent for Surgical or Diagnostic Instrument

A physician may patent a surgical or diagnostic instrument he or she has discovered or developed. The laws governing patents are based on the sound doctrine that one is entitled to protect one's discovery. (V, VII)

Issued prior to April 1977.

9.095 Patenting of Medical Procedures

A physician has the ethical responsibility not only to learn from but also to contribute to the total store of scientific knowledge when possible. Physicians should strive to advance medical science and make their advances known to patients, colleagues and the public. This obligation provides not merely incentive but imperative to innovate and share the ensuing advances. The patenting of medical procedures poses substantial risks to the effective practice of medicine by limiting the availability of new procedures to patients and should be condemned on this basis. Accordingly, it is unethical for physicians to seek, secure or enforce patents on medical procedures. (V, VII)

Issued June 1996 based on the report "Ethical Issues in the Patenting of Medical Procedures," adopted June 1995.

9.10   Peer Review

Medical society ethics committees, hospital credentials and utilization committees, and other forms of peer review have been long established by organized medicine to scrutinize physicians' professional conduct. At least to some extent, each of these types of peer review can be said to impinge upon the absolute professional freedom of physicians. They are, nonetheless, recognized and accepted. They are necessary and committees performing such work act ethically as long as principles of due process (Opinion 9.05) are observed. They balance the physician's right to exercise medical judgment freely with the obligation to do so wisely and temperately. (II, III, VII)

Issued prior to April 1977.

Updated June 1994.

9.11   The previous opinion 9.11, **Physician Impairment**, issued December 1986, was deleted in June 1994.

9.11   Ethics Committees in Health Care Institutions

The following guidelines have been developed to aid in the establishment and functioning of ethics committees in hospitals and other health care institutions that may choose to form such committees.
(1) Ethics committees in health care institutions should be educational and advisory in purpose. Generally, the function of the ethics committee should be to consider and assist in resolving unusual, complicated ethical problems involving issues that affect the care and treatment of patients within the health care institution. Recommendations of the ethics committee should impose no obligation for acceptance on the part of the institution, its governing board, medical staff, attending physician, or other persons. However, it should be expected that the recommendations of a dedicated ethics committee will receive serious consideration by decision makers.
(2) The size of the committee should be consistent with the needs of the institution but not so large as to be unwieldy. Committee members should be selected on the basis of their concern for the welfare of the sick and infirm, their interest in ethical matters, and their reputation in the community and among their peers for integrity and mature judgment. Experience as a member of hospital or medical society committees concerned with ethical conduct or quality assurance should be considered in selecting ethics committee members. Committee members should not have other responsibilities that are likely to prove incompatible with their duties as members of the ethics

committee. Preferably, a majority of the committee should consist of physicians, nurses, and other health care providers. In hospitals, medical staff bylaws should delineate the functions of the committee, general qualifications for membership, and manner of selection of members, in accordance with these guidelines.

(3) The functions of the ethics committee should be confined exclusively to ethical matters. The Code of Medical Ethics of the American Medical Association is recommended for the guidance of ethics committees in making their own recommendations. The matters to be considered by the committee should consist of ethical subjects that a majority of its members may choose to discuss on its own initiative, matters referred to it by the executive commitee of the organized medical staff or by the governing board of the institution, or appropriate requests from patients, families, or health care providers.

(4) In denominational health care institutions or those operated by religious orders, the recommendations of the ethics committee may be anticipated to be consistent with published religious tenets and principles. Where particular religious beliefs are to be taken into consideration in the committee's recommendations, this fact should be publicized to physicians, patients, and others concerned with the committee's recommendations.

(5) In its deliberations and communication of recommendations, the procedures followed by the ethics committee should comply with institutional and ethical policies for preserving the confidentiality of information regarding patients.

(6) Committee members should be prepared to meet on short notice and to render their recommendations in a timely and prompt fashion in accordance with the demands of the situation and the issues involved. (II, IV, VII)

Issued June 1994 based on the report "Guidelines for Ethics Committees in Health Care Institutions," adopted December 1984 (JAMA. 1985; 253: 2698-2699).

9.115 Ethics Consultations

Ethics consultations may be called to clarify ethical issues without reference to a particular case, facilitate discussion of an ethical dilemma in a particular case, or resolve an ethical dispute. The consultation mechanism may be through an ethics committee, a subset of the committee, individual consultants or consultation teams. The following guidelines are offered with respect to these services:

(1) All hospitals and other health care institutions should provide access to ethics consultation services. Health care facilities without ethics committees or consultation services should develop flexible, efficient mechanisms of ethics review that divide the burden of committee functioning among collaborating health care facilities.

(2) Institutions offering ethics consultation services must appreciate the complexity of the task, recognizing the potential for harm as well as benefit, and act responsibly. This includes true institutional support for the service.

(3) Ethics consultation services require a serious investment of time and effort by the individuals involved. Members should include either individuals with extensive formal training and experience in clinical ethics or individ-

uals who have made a substantial commitment over several years to gain sufficient knowledge, skills, and understanding of the complexity of clinical ethics. A wide variety of background training is preferable, including such fields as philosophy, religion, medicine, and law.

(4) Explicit structural standards should be developed and consistently followed. These should include developing a clear description of the consultation service's role and determining which types of cases will be addressed, how the cases will be referred to the service, whether the service will provide recommendations or simply function as a forum for discussion, and whether recommendations are binding or advisory.

(5) Explicit procedural standards should be developed and consistently followed. These should include establishing who must be involved in the consultation process and how notification, informed consent, confidentiality and case write-ups will be handled.

(6) In general, patient and staff informed consent may be presumed for ethics consultation. However, patients and families should be given the opportunity not to participate in discussions either formally, through the institutional process, or informally.

(7) In those cases where the patient or family has chosen not to participate in the consultation process, the final recommendations of the consultant(s) should be tempered.

(8) In general, ethics consultation services, like social services, should be financed by the institution.

(9) A consultation service should be careful not to take on more than it can handle, *i.e.* the complexity of the role should correspond to the level of sophistication of the service and the resources it has available. As a result, some services may offer only information and education, others a forum for discussion but not advice, others might serve a mediation role, and some might handle even administrative or organizational ethics issues. (IV, V)

Issued June 1998 based on the report "Ethics Consultations," adopted December 1997.

9.12 Patient-Physician Relationship: Respect for Law and Human Rights

The creation of the patient-physician relationship is contractual in nature. Generally, both the physician and the patient are free to enter into or decline the relationship. A physician may decline to undertake the care of a patient whose medical condition is not within the physician's current competence. However, physicians who offer their services to the public may not decline to accept patients because of race, color, religion, national origin, sexual orientation, or any other basis that would constitute invidious discrimination. Furthermore, physicians who are obligated under pre-existing contractual arrangements may not decline to accept patients as provided by those arrangements. (I, III, V, VI)

Issued July 1986.

Updated June 1994.

9.121 Racial Disparities in Health Care

Disparities in medical care based on immutable characteristics such as race must be avoided. Whether such disparities in health care are caused by treatment decisions, differences in income and education, sociocultural factors, or failures by the medical profession, they are unjustifiable and must be eliminated. Physicians should examine their own practices to ensure that racial prejudice does not affect clinical judgment in medical care. (I, IV)

Issued March 1992 based on the report "Black-White Disparities in Health Care," adopted December 1989 (JAMA. 1990; 263: 2344-2346).

Updated June 1994.

9.122 Gender Disparities in Health Care

A patient's gender plays an appropriate role in medical decision making when biological differences between the sexes are considered. However, some data suggest that gender bias may be playing a role in medical decision making. Social attitudes, including stereotypes, prejudices and other evaluations based on gender role expectations may play themselves out in a variety of subtle ways. Physicians must ensure that gender is not used inappropriately as a consideration in clinical decision making. Physicians should examine their practices and attitudes for influence of social or cultural biases which could be inadvertently affecting the delivery of medical care.

Research on health problems that affect both genders should include male and female subjects, and results of medical research done solely on males should not be generalized to females without evidence that results apply to both sexes. Medicine and society in general should ensure that resources for medical research should be distributed in a manner which promotes the health of both sexes to the greatest extent possible. (I, IV)

Issued March 1992 based on the report "Gender Disparities in Clinical Decision Making," adopted December 1990 (JAMA. 1991; 266: 559-562).

Updated June 1994.

9.13 Physicians and Infectious Diseases

A physician who knows that he or she has an infectious disease, which if contracted by the patient would pose a significant risk to the patient, should not engage in any activity that creates a significant risk of transmission of that disease to the patient. The precautions taken to prevent the transmission of a contagious disease to a patient should be appropriate to the seriousness of the disease and must be particularly stringent in the case of a disease that is potentially fatal. (I, IV)

Issued August 1989.

Updated June 1996 and June 1999.

9.131 HIV-Infected Patients and Physicians

A physician may not ethically refuse to treat a patient whose condition is within the physician's current realm of competence solely because the patient is seropositive for HIV. Persons who are seropositive should not be subjected to discrimination based on fear or prejudice.

When physicians are unable to provide the services required by an HIV-infected patient, they should make appropriate referrals to those physicians or facilities equipped to provide such services.

A physician who knows that he or she is seropositive should not engage in any activity that creates a significant risk of transmission of the disease to others. A physician who has HIV disease or who is seropositive should consult colleagues as to which activities the physician can pursue without creating a risk to patients. (I, II, IV)

Issued March 1992 based on the report "Ethical Issues in the Growing AIDS Crisis," adopted December 1987 (JAMA. 1988; 259: 1360-1361).

Updated June 1996 and June 1998.

9.132 Health Care Fraud and Abuse

The following guidelines encourage physicians to play a key role in identifying and preventing fraud:
(1) Physicians must renew their commitment to Section II of the AMA's Principles of Medical Ethics which states that "a physician shall deal honestly with patients and colleagues, and strive to expose those physicians deficient in character, competence, or who engage in fraud or deception."
(2) Physicians should make no intentional misrepresentations to increase the level of payment they receive or to secure non-covered health benefits for their patients. (II)

Issued June 1998 based on the report "Health Care Fraud and Abuse," adopted December 1997.

10.00 Opinions on the Patient-Physician Relationship

10.01 Fundamental Elements of the Patient-Physician Relationship

From ancient times, physicians have recognized that the health and well-being of patients depends upon a collaborative effort between physician and patient. Patients share with physicians the responsibility for their own health care. The patient-physician relationship is of greatest benefit to patients when they bring medical problems to the attention of their physicians in a timely fashion, provide information about their medical condition to the best of their ability, and work with their physicians in a mutually respectful alliance. Physicians can best contribute to this alliance by serving as their patients' advocate and by fostering these rights:

(1) The patient has the right to receive information from physicians and to discuss the benefits, risks, and costs of appropriate treatment alternatives. Patients should receive guidance from their physicians as to the optimal course of action. Patients are also entitled to obtain copies or summaries of their medical records, to have their questions answered, to be advised of potential conflicts of interest that their physicians might have, and to receive independent professional opinions.

(2) The patient has the right to make decisions regarding the health care that is recommended by his or her physician. Accordingly, patients may accept or refuse any recommended medical treatment.

(3) The patient has the right to courtesy, respect, dignity, responsiveness, and timely attention to his or her needs.

(4) The patient has the right to confidentiality. The physician should not reveal confidential communications or information without the consent of the patient, unless provided for by law or by the need to protect the welfare of the individual or the public interest.

(5) The patient has the right to continuity of health care. The physician has an obligation to cooperate in the coordination of medically indicated care with other health care providers treating the patient. The physician may not discontinue treatment of a patient as long as further treatment is medically indicated, without giving the patient reasonable assistance and sufficient opportunity to make alternative arrangements for care.

(6) The patient has a basic right to have available adequate health care. Physicians, along with the rest of society, should continue to work toward this goal. Fulfillment of this right is dependent on society providing resources so that no patient is deprived of necessary care because of an inability to pay for the care. Physicians should continue their traditional assumption of a part of the responsibility for the medical care of those who

cannot afford essential health care. Physicians should advocate for patients in dealing with third parties when appropriate.

Issued June 1992 based on the report "Fundamental Elements of the Patient-Physician Relationship," adopted June 1990.

Updated 1993.

10.02 Patient Responsibilities

It has long been recognized that successful medical care requires an ongoing collaborative effort between patients and physicians. Physician and patient are bound in a partnership that requires both individuals to take an active role in the healing process. Such a partnership does not imply that both partners have identical responsibilities or equal power. While physicians have the responsibility to provide health care services to patients to the best of their ability, patients have the responsibility to communicate openly, to participate in decisions about the diagnostic and treatment recommendations, and to comply with the agreed upon treatment program.

Like patients' rights, patients' responsibilities are derived from the principle of autonomy. The principle of patient autonomy holds that an individual's physical, emotional, and psychological integrity should be respected and upheld. This principle also recognizes the human capacity to self-govern and choose a course of action from among different alternative options. Autonomous, competent patients assert some control over the decisions which direct their health care. With that exercise of self-governance and free choice comes a number of responsibilities.

(1) Good communication is essential to a successful patient-physician relationship. To the extent possible, patients have a responsibility to be truthful and to express their concerns clearly to their physicians.

(2) Patients have a responsibility to provide a complete medical history, to the extent possible, including information about past illnesses, medications, hospitalizations, family history of illness and other matters relating to present health.

(3) Patients have a responsibility to request information or clarification about their health status or treatment when they do not fully understand what has been described.

(4) Once patients and physicians agree upon the goals of therapy and a treatment plan, patients have a responsibility to cooperate with that treatment plan. Compliance with physician instructions is often essential to public and individual safety. Patients also have a responsibility to disclose whether previously agreed upon treatments are being followed and to indicate when they would like to reconsider the treatment plan.

(5) Patients generally have a responsibility to meet their financial obligations with regard to medical care or to discuss financial hardships with their physicians. Patients should be cognizant of the costs associated with using a limited resource like health care and try to use medical resources judiciously.

(6) Patients should discuss end-of-life decisions with their physicians and make their wishes known. Such a discussion might also include writing an advanced directive.

(7) Patients should be committed to health maintenance through health-enhancing behavior. Illness can often be prevented by a healthy lifestyle, and patients should take personal responsibility when they are able to avert the development of disease.

(8) Patients should also have an active interest in the effects of their conduct on others and refrain from behavior that unreasonably places the health of others at risk. Patients should inquire as to the means and likelihood of infectious disease transmission and act upon that information which can best prevent further transmission.

(9) Patients should discuss organ donation with their physicians and, if donation is desired, make applicable provisions. Patients who are part of an organ allocation system and await needed transplant should not try to go outside of or manipulate the system. A fair system of allocation should be answered with public trust and an awareness of limited resources.

(10) Patients should not initiate or participate in fraudulent health care and should report illegal or unethical behavior by physicians and other providers to the appropriate medical societies, licensing boards, or law enforcement authorities.

Issued June 1994 based on the report "Patient Responsibilities," adopted June 1993.

Updated June 1998.

10.03   Patient-Physician Relationship in the Context of Work-Related and Independent Medical Examinations

When a physician is responsible for performing an isolated assessment of an individual's health or disability for an employer, business, or insurer, a limited patient-physician relationship should be considered to exist. Both "Industry Employed Physicians" (IEPs), who are employed by businesses or insurance companies for the purpose of conducting medical examinations, and "Independent Medical Examiners" (IMEs), who are independent contractors providing medical examinations within the realm of their specialty, may perform such medical examinations.

Despite their ties to a third party, the responsibilities of IEPs and IMEs are in some basic respects very similar to those of other physicians. IEPs and IMEs have the same obligations as physicians in other contexts to:

(1) Evaluate objectively the patient's health or disability. In order to maintain objectivity, IEPs and IMEs should not be influenced by the preferences of the patient-employee, employer, or insurance company when making a diagnosis during a work-related or independent medical examination.

(2) Maintain patient confidentiality as outlined by Opinion 5.09, Industry Employed Physicians and Independent Medical Examiners.

(3) Disclose fully potential or perceived conflicts of interest. The physician should inform the patient about the terms of the agreement between

himself or herself and the third party as well as the fact that he or she is acting as an agent of that entity. This should be done at the outset of the examination, before health information is gathered from the patient-employee. Before the physician proceeds with the exam, he or she should ensure to the extent possible that the patient understands the physician's unaltered ethical obligations, as well as the differences that exist between the physician's role in this context and the physician's traditional fiduciary role.

IEPs and IMEs are responsible for administering an objective medical evaluation but not for monitoring patients' health over time, treating patients, or fulfilling many other duties traditionally held by physicians. Consequently, a limited patient-physician relationship should be considered to exist during isolated assessments of an individual's health or disability for an employer, business, or insurer.

The physician has a responsibility to inform the patient about important health information or abnormalities that he or she discovers during the course of the examination. In addition, the physician should ensure to the extent possible that the patient understands the problem or diagnosis. Furthermore, when appropriate, the physician should suggest that the patient seek care from a qualified physician and, if requested, provide reasonable assistance in securing follow-up care. (I)

Issued December 1999 based on the report "Patient-Physician Relationship in the Context of Work-Related and Independent Medical Examinations," adopted June 1999.

American Medical Association
Constitution and Bylaws
Council on Ethical and Judicial Affairs

Authority

The Council on Ethical and Judicial Affairs is the judicial authority of the American Medical Association and its decision shall be final.

Functions

The functions of the Council on Ethical and Judicial Affairs are:
- To interpret the Principles of Medical Ethics of the American Medical Association.
- To interpret the Constitution, Bylaws and rules of the Association.
- To investigate general ethical conditions and all matters pertaining to the relations of physicians to one another or to the public, and make recommendations to the House of Delegates or the constituent associations.
- To receive appeals filed by applicants who allege that they, because of color, creed, race, religion, ethnic origin, national origin, or sex, have been unfairly denied membership in a component and/or constituent association, to determine the facts in the case, and to report the findings to the House of Delegates. If the Council determines that the allegations are indeed true, it shall admonish, censure, or in the event of repeated violations, recommend to the House of Delegates that the constituent association involved be declared to be no longer a constituent member of the American Medical Association.
- To request the President to appoint investigating juries to which it may refer complaints or evidences of unethical conduct which in its judgment are of greater than local concern. Such investigative juries, if probable cause for action be shown, shall submit formal charges to the President, who shall appoint a prosecutor to prosecute such charges against the accused before the Council on Ethical and Judicial Affairs in the name and on behalf of the American Medical Association. The Council may acquit, admonish, suspend or expel the accused.
- To approve applications and nominate candidates for affiliate membership as otherwise provided for in 1.141 of these Bylaws.

Original Jurisdiction

The Council on Ethical and Judicial Affairs shall have original jurisdiction in:
- All questions involving membership.

- All controversies arising under this Constitution and Bylaws and under the Principles of Medical Ethics to which the American Medical Association is a party.
- Controversies between two or more state associations or their members and between a constituent association and a component society or societies of another state association or associations or their members.

Appellate Jurisdiction

The Council on Ethical and Judicial Affairs shall have appellate jurisdiction in questions of law and procedure but not of fact in all cases which arise:

A. Between a constituent association and one or more of its component societies.
B. Between component societies of the same constituent association.
C. Between a member or members and the component society to which said member or members belong following an appeal to the member's constituent association.
D. Between members of different component societies of the same constituent association following a decision by the constituent association.

Appeal Mechanisms

Notice of appeal shall be filed with the Council on Ethical and Judicial Affairs within thirty (30) days of the date of the decision by the state association and the appeal shall be perfected within sixty (60) days thereof; provided, however, that the Council on Ethical and Judicial Affairs, for what it considers good and sufficient cause, may grant an additional thirty (30) days for perfecting the appeal.

Membership

The Council on Ethical and Judicial Affairs shall consist of nine Active members of the American Medical Association, including one Resident Physician member and one Medical Student member. Members elected to the Council on Ethical and Judicial Affairs shall resign all other positions held by them in the Association upon their election to the Council. No member, while serving on the Council on Ethical and Judicial Affairs, shall be a delegate or an alternate delegate to the House of Delegates, or a General Officer of the Association, or serve on any other council, committee or as Representative to or Governing Council Member of a Special Section of the American Medical Association.

Limit on Medical Student Participation

The Medical Student member of the Council shall have the right to participate fully in the work of the Council, except that in disciplinary matters and in matters relating to membership the Medical Student member shall participate only if a medical student is the subject of the disciplinary matter or is the applicant for membership.

Nomination and Election

The members of the Council shall be elected by the House of Delegates on nomination by the President. State Medical Associations, National Medical Specialty Societies, Special Sections of the AMA, and other organizations represented in the AMA House of Delegates, and members of the Board of Trustees may submit the names and qualifications of candidates for consideration by the President.

Term of Service

Members of the Council on Ethical and Judicial Affairs shall be elected by the House of Delegates for the following terms of office:

- The Medical Student member of the Council shall be elected for a term of two years, provided that if the Medical Student member ceases to be enrolled in an approved medical school or in an osteopathic medical school approved by an appropriate accrediting agency at any time prior to the expiration of the term for which the Medical Student member was elected, the service of such Medical Student member on the Council shall thereupon terminate, and the position shall be declared vacant. The Council shall determine the voting privileges of the Medical Student member for each term of service.

- The Resident Physician Member of the Council shall be elected for a term of three years provided that if the Resident member ceases to be in an approved training program at any time prior to the expiration of the term for which the Resident Physician member was elected, the service of such Resident member on the Council shall thereupon terminate, and the position shall be declared vacant. The Resident Physician member shall have the right to vote in all matters in which said member participates under the rules of the Council.

- All other members of the Council shall be elected by the House of Delegates for a term of seven years, so arranged that at each Annual Convention the term of one member shall expire.

Tenure

Members of the Council on Ethical and Judicial Affairs shall serve only one term, except that the Resident Physician member and the Medical Student member shall be eligible to serve for two terms. A member elected to serve an unexpired term shall not be regarded as having served a term unless such member has served at least half of said term.

Vacancies

Members Other Than The Resident Member. Any vacancy among the members of the Council on Ethical and Judicial Affairs other than the Resident member shall be filled at the next meeting of the House of Delegates. The new member shall be elected by the House of Delegates, on nomination by the President, for the remainder of the unexpired term.

Resident Member. If the Resident Physician member of the Council is unable, for any reason, to complete the term for which he or she was elected, the remainder of the term shall be deemed to have expired. The successor shall be elected by the House of Delegates at its next meeting, on nomination by the President, for a term to expire at the conclusion of the third Annual Meeting of the House of Delegates following the meeting at which said Resident was elected.

Rules of the Council on Ethical and Judicial Affairs

Rule I. Administration

A. **Meetings.** The Council on Ethical and Judicial Affairs will meet during the Annual and Interim Meetings of the American Medical Association. Other meetings of the Council may be called, on reasonable notice, by the Chair of the Council; or they shall be called, on reasonable notice, by the Executive Vice President of the American Medical Association on the written request of at least five members of the Council.

B. **Chair and Vice-Chair.** At the reorganization meeting of the Council which shall be held during each Annual Meeting of the AMA after election of members to the Council, the Council on Ethical and Judicial Affairs shall elect a chair and a vice-chair from among its members except that the resident physician and medical student members of the Council shall not be eligible to serve as chair or vice-chair. The chair and the vice-chair shall retain the right to vote on all matters. No member of the Council shall serve more than two consecutive years as chair or two consecutive years as vice-chair.

The chair and vice-chair to be so elected shall be elected on separate, secret ballots. The balloting and voting for chair shall be completed and a chair elected before the balloting and voting for the vice-chair begins. A majority vote of the entire Council shall be required to so elect either a chair or a vice-chair, with balloting and voting to be repeated, if necessary, until a member is elected to each position.

In the event that the position of chair becomes permanently vacant for any reason during the term of the then currently serving chair, the then currently serving vice-chair shall immediately assume the position of chair for the remainder of the term. A new vice-chair shall then be elected by secret ballot at the ensuing meeting of the Council to serve the remainder of the immediately preceding vice-chair's term. A majority vote of the entire Council, as then constituted, shall be required to so elect a vice-chair, with balloting and voting to be repeated, if necessary, until a member is elected vice-chair. The serving of the balance of a term as chair or vice-chair due to such a vacancy shall not be counted in determining whether a member of the Council has served more than two consecutive years as chair or two consecutive years as vice-chair.

In the event that the position of vice-chair becomes permanently vacant for any reason during the term of the then currently serving vice-chair, a new vice-chair shall be elected by secret ballot at the ensuing meeting of the Council to serve the remainder of the immediately preceding vice-chair's term. A majority vote of the entire Council, as then constituted, shall be required to so elect a vice-chair, with balloting and voting to be repeated, if necessary, until a member is elected vice-chair. The serving of the balance of a term as vice-chair due to such a vacancy shall not be counted in determining whether a member of the Council has served more than two consecutive years as vice-chair.

C. **Student Members.** The medical student member of the Council shall participate as a regular member in the interpretation of the Principles of Medical Ethics of the American Medical Association, the interpretation of the Constitution, Bylaws and rules of the Association, and the investigation of general ethical conditions and all matters pertaining to the relations of physicians to one another or to the public. The medical student member of the Council shall have the right to participate in disciplinary matters and in matters relating to membership only if a medical student is the subject of the disciplinary matter or is the applicant for membership.

D. **Quorum.** A majority of the members of the Council on Ethical and Judicial Affairs eligible to vote on a matter shall constitute a quorum and shall be required to adopt any action.

E. **Confidentiality.** All matters under consideration for adoption by the Council shall be treated as confidential until adopted by the Council.

Rule II. Applications for Membership

A. **Active Membership.** Applications for membership in the American Medical Association will be considered by the Council on Ethical and Judicial Affairs at any meeting upon presentation of the applications by the Executive Vice President of the Association.

B. **Affiliate Membership.** Applications for affiliate membership submitted by (1) physicians in foreign countries who have attained distinction in medicine and who are members of the national medical society or such other organization as will verify their professional credentials, (2) American physicians located in foreign countries or possessions of the United States and engaged in medical missionary, educational or philanthropic endeavors, (3) dentists who hold the degree of D.D.S. or D.M.D., who are members of the American Dental Association and their state and local dental societies, (4) pharmacists who are active members of the American Pharmaceutical Association, (5) teachers of medicine or of the sciences allied to medicine who are citizens of the United States and are ineligible for active or associate membership, or (6) individuals engaged in scientific endeavors allied to medicine and others who have attained distinction in their fields of endeavor who are not otherwise eligible for membership, may be considered at any meeting of the Council on presentation of the applications by the Executive Vice President of the Association. The Council will consider and approve only those applications which are accompanied by a statement of a responsible and qualified individual attesting to the requirements set forth above. (Employees of the AMA or any AMA affiliate or subsidiary may be eligible affiliate members under subsection (6). They must have five years of employment at the AMA, affiliate, or subsidiary and their distinction in their field of endeavor must be certified by an AMA Senior Vice President, or if the employee is a Senior Vice President, the Executive Vice President.)

C. **Refusal of Approval.** An applicant for membership in the American Medical Association whose application has not been approved by the Council on Ethical and Judicial Affairs will be promptly notified of such fact.

Rule III. Physicians Denied Membership in Component or Constituent Associations

Pursuant to 6.4024 of the Bylaws, any physician whose application for membership in a component and/or constituent association has allegedly been denied unfairly because of color, creed, race, religion, ethnic origin, national origin, or sex may appeal to the Council on Ethical and Judicial Affairs.

The Council shall determine the facts in the case and report the findings to the House of Delegates. If the Council determines that the allegations are indeed true, it shall admonish, censure or, in the event of repeated violations, recommend to the House of Delegates that the state association involved be declared to be no longer a constituent member of the American Medical Association.

Proceedings for such determination shall be initiated by a written statement. Such statement shall: (1) identify the parties to the case, (2) show that the appellant has exhausted remedies made available by the constitution and bylaws of the component society and the state association, and (3) include a concise factual resume of the case in sufficient detail to enable the Council to ascertain the facts. The appellant should also furnish such other information as may be requested by or helpful to the Council in determining the facts.

Rule IV. Original Controversies

Original proceedings before the Council on Ethical and Judicial Affairs shall be initiated by a written statement. Such statement shall include information (1) identifying the parties to the controversy, including membership affiliations, if applicable, and (2) explaining the nature of the controversy, setting forth the provisions of the Constitution, Bylaws, Rules, or Principles of Medical Ethics concerned.

Rule V. Appeals

Appellate proceedings before the Council on Ethical and Judicial Affairs shall be perfected by a written statement of appeal. Such statement shall include information (1) identifying the parties to the case and indicating membership affiliations when appropriate, (2) showing that the appellant has exhausted remedies made available by the constitution and bylaws of the component society and the state association, and (3) describing the error of law or procedure which is believed to have occurred during the proceedings. The statement shall also include a concise, factual resume of the case. Appellant shall submit with the statement the charges, complaints, findings, opinions, and decisions previously entered in the case.

Rule VI. Interpretation of the Constitution, Bylaws, Rules and Principles of Medical Ethics of the American Medical Association

A. **Requests for Interpretation.** Requests for interpretation of the Constitution, Bylaws, Rules, or Principles of Medical Ethics of the Association shall be in writing and shall describe the matter to be interpreted in sufficient detail to enable the members of the Council on Ethical and Judicial Affairs to evaluate the request in all its aspects.

B. **Interpretations Initiated by the Council.** The Council on Ethical and Judicial Affairs on its own motion, may render an opinion concerning the interpretation or application of the Constitution, Bylaws, Rules, or Principles of Medical Ethics of the Association and may, on its own motion, consider and decide the constitutionality and validity of all rules and regulations adopted by Councils and Committees of the Association pursuant to the Bylaws of the Association.

C. **Discretionary Power.** The Council on Ethical and Judicial Affairs may, in its own discretion, refuse to consider requests for interpretation of the Principles of Medical Ethics which in the opinion of the Council should be resolved by a component society or a state association. Requests for interpretation of the Principles of Medical Ethics which are not of national interest and relate to the observance of local customs and ideals may be readdressed to the component society or constituent association primarily responsible for knowledge of the requirements of such local customs and recognized ideals.

Rule VII. Jurisdiction

The Council on Ethical and Judicial Affairs may, on its own motion or on the motion of any party, determine the question of jurisdiction at any stage of the proceedings.

Rule VIII. Additional Statements and Record

After a statement has been submitted to the Council on Ethical and Judicial Affairs with the intention of initiating an action, all other parties in interest shall have the right to submit a statement on their behalf. Such statement shall be filed within thirty (30) days after the filing of the initiating statement unless additional time is granted by the Council.

The Council on Ethical and Judicial Affairs may thereafter require the parties to submit such transcripts of testimony, records, written statements supporting their contentions, or other material as the Council may deem necessary.

Rule IX. Hearings

A. **Notice of Hearings.** The Council may in its discretion determine whether a hearing is necessary or advisable. The Council will designate the time and place for all hearings, giving reasonable notice thereof to all parties.

B. **Attendance.** Attendance at hearings may be limited to the members of the Council on Ethical and Judicial Affairs, the staff, witnesses, if any, the parties, and counsel, who may speak in their behalf. Should any party to the controversy fail to appear, the Council may in its discretion continue, dismiss, or decide the matter.

C. **Evidence and Argument.** The Council on Ethical and Judicial Affairs will not be bound by technical rules of evidence usually employed in legal proceedings but may accept any evidence it deems appropriate and pertinent.

In any appeal case the review, if any, of the evidence will be limited to the evidence presented in the proceedings before the component society and constituent association or appropriate committee, board, or group thereof; provided, however, that in the event the Council is of the opinion such evidence is inadequate to determine the question of law or procedure presented, the Council, on its own motion or on the suggestion of any party, may require the production of additional evidence before the Council or refer the matter to the appropriate body for additional evidence.

In matters other than appeal cases, the Council will grant the parties the right to present evidence to the extent the Council believes appropriate to the particular matter in controversy.

In all hearings, the Council, within reasonable limitations, will allow oral argument.

D. **Record.** In hearings of original controversies, appeals, and in other proceedings, a transcript may be made at the discretion of the Council.

Rule X. Opinions

All opinions or decisions of the Council on Ethical and Judicial Affairs shall be in writing. Copies of the opinion or decision and the dissent, if any, will be filed as a part of the record and furnished to all the parties involved.

Rule XI. Filing and Copies

Ten (10) copies of all documents shall be submitted to the Secretary of the Council on Ethical and Judicial Affairs. One copy of each document shall be submitted at the same time to each of the other parties to the controversy.

Rule XII. AMA Membership Applications

A. Section 1.121 of the AMA Bylaws provides that Active Direct members shall be admitted to membership upon application to the Executive Vice President of the AMA, provided that there is no disapproval by the AMA Council on Ethical and Judicial Affairs. Section 1.1212 of the AMA Bylaws provides that objections to applicants for Active Direct Membership will be referred to the Council for prompt disposition pursuant to the rules of the Council. Section 1.111 of the AMA Bylaws provides that Active Constituent members shall be admitted to membership upon certification by the secretary of the constituent association to the Executive Vice President of the AMA provided that there is no disapproval by the AMA Council on Ethical and Judicial Affairs.

B. In reviewing applications for AMA membership, the Council on Ethical and Judicial Affairs shall consider information contained in the application, information from other available sources and objections raised in response to notification of the state medical association or associations in the jurisdiction or jurisdictions in which the applicant practices. The Council may consider information pertaining to the character, ethics, professional status and professional activities of the applicant. Any significant misstatements or omissions from the application shall constitute cause for denial of AMA membership.

C. Following review of the application for AMA membership and related information, the applicant shall be notified of allegations, which if true, would justify denial of AMA membership. The applicant shall have thirty (30) days following receipt of the notice in which to file a written response. Failure of the applicant to respond within the thirty (30) day period waives any further consideration of the application. The Council on Ethical and Judicial Affairs shall consider any written response and determine whether additional information is needed to dispose of the matter in a fair and equitable manner.

D. If additional information is needed to resolve disputed issues of fact or the Council on Ethical and Judicial Affairs finds cause for disapproving an application, the applicant shall be notified in writing of the disputed issues of fact or reasons for disapproval and shall have thirty (30) days following receipt of the notice to request a hearing. Failure to request a hearing within the thirty (30) day period waives any further consideration of the application.

E. If the applicant submits a written request for a hearing, the Council on Ethical and Judicial Affairs shall notify the applicant of the date, place and time of the hearing and shall provide the applicant with a copy of these rules. Notice shall also be sent to anyone who submitted written objections to AMA membership by the applicant, informing them of the right, within seven (7) days after the date of the notice, to request to appear at their own expense to present evidence in support of the objections or refute evidence presented by the applicant. No objector shall have the right to cross-examine the applicant or any witnesses.

F. The Council on Ethical and Judicial Affairs shall not be bound by technical legal rules of evidence and may accept any evidence or information deemed reliable or relevant. The applicant shall not be required to, but may be accompanied by legal counsel and either the applicant or legal counsel may cross-examine any witnesses who appear in opposition to the applicant's application for AMA membership.

G. If a written transcript is made of the hearing, any party requesting a copy shall have it made available at his or her own expense.

H. The Council on Ethical and Judicial Affairs shall, within thirty (30) days after the hearing, notify the applicant and anyone who appeared at the hearing, of its decision.

I. If the decision is to deny membership, the applicant may reapply for membership after one year following the date of the decision.

Rule XIII. Discipline

Section 1.20 of the Bylaws provides that a member may retain membership only as long as the provisions of the Constitution and Bylaws and Principles of Medical Ethics of the American Medical Association are complied with. Sections 1.621, 6.401, and 6.4022 of the Bylaws provide that the Council on Ethical and Judicial Affairs, after due notice and hearing, may censure, place on probation, suspend or expel any active direct, associate, affiliate or honorary member of the AMA for an infraction of the Constitution and Bylaws or for a violation of the Principles of Medical Ethics of the AMA. Section 1.611 provides that the Council on Ethical and Judicial Affairs, after due notice and hearing, may censure, suspend or expel an active constituent association, for an infraction of the Constitution and Bylaws or for a violation of the Principles of Medical Ethics of the AMA. In addition, the AMA may take disciplinary action with respect to an active constituent member's AMA membership (1) when a state medical association to which a member belongs requests the AMA to take such action; or (2) when, at the request of the AMA, a state association to which the member belongs consents to such action. Section 6.4025 of the Bylaws provides that the Council on Ethical and Judicial Affairs may request the President of the Association to appoint investigating juries to which the Council may refer complaints or evidences of unethical conduct which, in its judgment, are of greater than local concern. The following Rules of Procedure, respecting notice of charges and the conduct of hearings before the Council, are based upon these Sections of the Bylaws.

A. **Statement of Charges**. The statement of charges shall allege in writing an infraction of the AMA's Constitution or Bylaws or a violation of the Principles of Medical Ethics of the AMA.

B. **Notice**. A copy of the statement of charges shall be sent to the member by registered or certified mail.

C. **Answer**. The member shall have sixty (60) days after receipt of the notice to file a written answer. The Council on Ethical and Judicial Affairs shall consider any written response and determine whether additional information is needed to dispose of the matter in a fair and equitable manner.

Failure of the member to respond within the sixty (60) day period shall constitute an admission of the allegations.

D. **Hearings**. Where additional information is needed to resolve disputed issues of fact or in cases where the Council on Ethical and Judicial Affairs finds cause for censuring, suspending or expelling a member, the member shall be notified in writing of the disputed issues of fact or reasons for censure, suspension or expulsion and shall have thirty (30) days following receipt of the notice to request a hearing. Failure to request a hearing within the thirty (30) day period waives the right to a hearing on the matter.

If the member submits a written request for a hearing, the Council on Ethical and Judicial Affairs shall notify the applicant of the date, place, and time of the hearing and shall provide the member with a copy of these rules. The member shall receive not less than thirty (30) days notice of the hearing. Notice shall also be sent to any state medical association to which an active constituent member belongs that has requested or consented to disciplinary action by the AMA; and such notice shall inform the state medical association of its right, within seven (7) days after the date of the notice, to request to appear at its own expense to present evidence in support of its allegation or refute evidence presented by the active constituent member, but the state medical association shall have no right to cross-examine the active constituent member or any witnesses.

The Council on Ethical and Judicial Affairs shall not be bound by technical legal rules of evidence and may accept any evidence or information deemed reliable or relevant. The General Counsel of the American Medical Association or her or his designee shall present the evidence against the member and may question the parties or their witnesses. The member shall not be required to, but may be accompanied by legal counsel and either the member or the member's legal counsel may cross-examine any witnesses who appear.

A written transcript shall be made of the hearing; any person requesting a copy shall have it made at his or her own expense.

E. **Decision**. The Council on Ethical and Judicial Affairs shall, within thirty (30) days after the hearing, notify the member of its decision and the reasons for any adverse decision. If the decision is to expel a member, he or she may reapply for membership after one year has elapsed from the date of the decision.

Rules of the Council on Ethical and Judicial Affairs in Original Jurisdiction Cases

Preamble

6.4025 of the Bylaws provides that the Council on Ethical and Judicial Affairs may request the President of the Association to appoint investigating juries to which the Council may refer complaints or evidences of unethical conduct which, in its judgment, are of greater than local concern.

The following Rules of Procedure, respecting notice of charges and the conduct of hearings before the Council on Ethical and Judicial Affairs are based upon this section of the Bylaws.

Investigating Jury

At the request of the Council on Ethical and Judicial Affairs, the President has appointed an investigating jury. Complaints or evidence of unethical conduct of greater than local concern will be submitted to this jury by the Council.

Institution of Proceedings

If after investigation a probable cause for action is shown, the investigating jury shall submit a statement of charges to the President. The President shall submit to the Council on Ethical and Judicial Affairs the statement of charges presented to him or her by the investigating jury for prosecution in the name and on behalf of the American Medical Association.

Statement of Charges

The statement of charges shall allege in writing an infraction of the AMA's Constitution or Bylaws or a violation of the Principles of Medical Ethics of the AMA. Exhibits may be attached.

Notice

A copy of the statement of charges shall be sent to the respondent physician by personal delivery or by registered or certified mail.

Answer

The respondent physician shall have thirty (30) days after personal delivery or mailing of the notice of statement of charges to file a written answer. If the respondent physician fails to file a written answer, the allegations shall be considered to be admitted.

Proceedings

The Chair of the Council on Ethical and Judicial Affairs shall designate one or more members of the Council to conduct a hearing on the statement of charges. This member or these members shall be known as the Hearing Officer.

Hearings shall be held at such reasonable time and place, designated by the Hearing Officer, as may be consistent with the nature of the proceedings and the convenience of the parties. The parties shall receive not less than fifteen (15) days of notice of the hearing.

The General Counsel of the American Medical Association or his or her designee shall prosecute the charges against the respondent physician.

Attendance at hearings may be limited to the members of the Council on Ethical and Judicial Affairs, the staff, witnesses, if any, the parties and counsel who may speak in their behalf.

The Hearing Officer or his counsel may question the parties and their witnesses. The Hearing Officer shall not be bound by technical rules of evidence usually employed in legal proceedings but may accept any evidence deemed appropriate and pertinent.

Should any party to the controversy fail to appear at the hearing, the Hearing Officer may, in his or her discretion, continue, dismiss or proceed with the hearing.

Findings and Conclusions

At the conclusion of the hearing, the Hearing Officer shall render a report in writing containing findings and conclusions and recommendations, if any. This report, together with a transcript of the proceedings, shall be submitted to the Council on Ethical and Judicial Affairs. A copy of the report shall be mailed to all parties of record.

Written Objections

Any party to the proceedings may submit written objections to the report to the Council on Ethical and Judicial Affairs. These objections must be submitted within twenty-one (21) days after the report has been submitted by the Hearing Officer to the Council on Ethical and Judicial Affairs.

Oral Argument

In addition to written objections, any party may request an opportunity to present oral arguments on its objections to the report of the Hearing Officer before the Council on Ethical and Judicial Affairs. This request must be made within twenty-one (21) days after the report has been submitted to the Council. The granting of oral arguments shall be discretionary with the Council. If granted, the parties shall be notified by the Council of the place and date for such oral argument; all parties shall be given opportunity to be heard and the time allotted to argument may be limited by the Council with due regard to the magnitude and complexities of the issues involved.

If any party fails to appear, the Council may continue or proceed with the oral argument.

Final Decision

The Council on Ethical and Judicial Affairs, including the member or members who serve as the Hearing Officer, shall render a final decision. A copy of that decision shall be mailed or otherwise served upon all parties.

Disciplinary Action

The Council on Ethical and Judicial Affairs shall have the authority to acquit, admonish, censure, or place on probation the accused physician or suspend or expel him or her from AMA membership as the facts may justify. This action shall be in accordance with the authority vested in the Council by 1.60, 6.401, 6.402 of the Bylaws.

Transcript

A written transcript shall be made of the proceedings and of the oral argument before the Council on Ethical and Judicial Affairs.

If any party to the controversy requests a copy of the transcript, it shall be made available to the party at the party's expense.

Filing of Copies

Ten (10) copies of all pleadings and exhibits shall be submitted to AMA Headquarters to the Chairman of the Council on Ethical and Judicial Affairs. One copy of each document shall be submitted at the same time to each of the other parties to the controversy.

Index